George Smith Heatley

The Stock-Owners' Guide

A handy Medical Treatise for every Man who owns an Ox or Cow

George Smith Heatley

The Stock-Owners' Guide
A handy Medical Treatise for every Man who owns an Ox or Cow

ISBN/EAN: 9783337183011

Printed in Europe, USA, Canada, Australia, Japan

Cover: Foto ©Lupo / pixelio.de

More available books at **www.hansebooks.com**

THE

STOCK-OWNERS' GUIDE

A HANDY MEDICAL TREATISE FOR EVERY
MAN WHO OWNS AN OX OR COW

BY

GEORGE S. HEATLEY
M.R.C.V.S.
AUTHOR OF 'THE HORSE-OWNERS' SAFEGUARD'

WILLIAM BLACKWOOD AND SONS
EDINBURGH AND LONDON
MDCCCLXXXIII

DEDICATED TO

ANDREW GILLON, ESQ. OF WALLHOUSE,

EX-CHAIRMAN OF THE

VETERINARY DEPARTMENT OF THE

HIGHLAND AND AGRICULTURAL SOCIETY OF SCOTLAND,

IN HONOUR OF HIS UNWEARIED EXERTIONS

AND SYMPATHETIC ZEAL,

DIRECTED TOWARDS THE DIFFUSION OF SCIENCE,

AND THE ALLEVIATION OF THE SUFFERINGS

OF THE LOWER ANIMALS,

BY HIS

HUMBLE AND OBEDIENT SERVANT

THE AUTHOR.

CONTENTS.

	PAGE
INTRODUCTION	1
DISEASES OF THE ACCESSORY ORGANS OF DIGESTION	49
DISEASES OF THE ORGANS OF RESPIRATION	56
DISEASES AFFECTING THE CIRCULATORY ORGANS	83
DISEASES OF THE URINARY ORGANS	88
DISEASES OF THE GENERATIVE ORGANS	92
DISEASES AFTER CALVING	97
DISEASES OF THE NERVOUS SYSTEM, MILK FEVER, ETC.	105
DISEASES OF THE BLOOD	119
DISEASES OF THE BONE	128
TUMOURS	132
DISEASES OF THE SKIN, ETC.	147
DISEASES OF THE EYE, ETC.	160

DISEASES OF CATTLE.

By the same Author.

In Crown 8vo, price 5s.

THE HORSE-OWNERS' SAFEGUARD: A HANDY MEDICAL GUIDE FOR EVERY MAN WHO OWNS A HORSE.

"We would strongly advise owners of horses to read the book for themselves. We presume that they will agree with us that 'The Horse-owners' Safeguard' is one of the best works of its kind published."—*Bell's Life in London.*

"If Mr. Heatley's volume is studied as it ought to be, equine animals would be protected from the pain of many ailments to which, without the interference of their owners, the race is naturally predisposed."—*Farmers' Gazette.*

"A most useful work on the management and treatment of horses . . . nearly every subject we can think of in connection with the horse is simply treated."—*Morning Post.*

"The volume will be found of great utility, and the author will be found an excellent and agreeable guide."—*Yorkshire Post.*

"To horse-owners, and those interested in horses, this is indeed a very valuable book."—*Dundee Advertiser.*

"Undoubtedly a most useful book for every one who owns a horse. . . . In many instances the life of a valuable animal might be saved by the owner having such a handy little volume as this by his side."—*Bell's Messenger.*

"The book can be most confidently recommended as a most valuable work for the large class to which it appeals."—*Perthshire Constitutional.*

"The book cannot fail to be useful to all who are entrusted with the management of horses."—*Derby Mercury.*

WILLIAM BLACKWOOD & SONS, EDINBURGH AND LONDON.

DISEASES OF CATTLE.

Introduction.

THE old adage that "a stitch in time saves nine" is equally applicable to the subjects that we are about to discuss.

The ox and cow are liable to many diseases from which the horse claims immunity; but in the former class of animals, disease, as a rule, requires a much longer time to develop; while it must be remembered that from the habits of the bovine race considerable difficulty is often experienced in detecting trouble, as the manifestations or symptoms of disease in them are in a great measure held in abeyance for several days; therefore the uninitiated may ignore or despise a characteristic sign that would at once put the cautious man on the alert. Our object, then, is to convey such information as will enable all who are interested to determine what is wrong, and to assist in its rectification as speedily as possible. We have all an incumbent duty to perform towards the lower animals, and there is none more worthy of our sympathy and help than the ox and cow, whose ailments we will now consider.

Description of Disease.

Disease may be said to consist of a deviation from the healthy standard either of function or of structure (or the opposite to health), and is a disturbance of function with alteration of structure of the living organism. It is also modified in different animals according to their organisation. For example, in the horse we have flatulent colic in the large intestines, because they contain a great quantity of fermentable food. In the ox we have hoven or distension of the first stomach, produced by the same cause; therefore the only difference betwixt hoven and flatulent colic is that they arise in separate regions of the internal abdominal cavity; the causes that were in operation to produce them being one and the same. But there is yet another consideration which must be recognised, and that is the peculiar and varied temperament of the different animals that claim our attention in health and disease. Again, cattle lay on fat readily, possess a large, sanguineous, plethoric system, and are more temperate, consequently diseases in them are developed less rapidly. The horse, on the other hand, has a very excitable nervous system, and is therefore rendered more susceptible to attack. Diseases are also geographically distributed, some being more prevalent in one district than in another. Again, animals of the same class, colour, and conformation are more susceptible to disease. They withstand disease variably; for inflammation of the bowels will destroy a horse in six hours, whereas in a cow the same disease will continue for a fortnight ere it produces death. This rule is indisputable in many other inflammatory affections, killing the horse in a few hours, whilst it takes days or weeks to cause death in the bovine race. Another question arises, How does disease kill or destroy life? Disease kills in one of two ways, that is, either by the suspension of the heart's action or by impeding respiration. This may be done suddenly or gradually, but nervous influences play a conspicuous part in both. Now a great many diseases consist in some change, either in the blood itself or some other fluid, by which the different tissues should be nourished and maintained; therefore it becomes imperative that we know something concerning the fluids of the body.

Now the fluids which enter the blood are of two kinds: first, those fluids which enter the blood for its nourishment and for the purpose of renewing it, the principle of which is chyle; secondly, those fluids which enter the blood and are carried out of the system, as those that proceed from the blood have again to enter the body. Those fluids, then, are divided into four classes:—

First, The excrementitious, or those that are of no more use to the animal economy, such as sweat, urine, &c.

Secondly, The recrementitious, or those fluids that, having been separated from the blood, are again returned to it, such as the *pancreatic, salivary*, and *gastric juices*.

Thirdly, The intermediate, or those fluids that are partly excrementitious and partly recrementitious, such as bile; and,

Fourthly, The special fluids, such as milk, &c.

These, then, are the fluids that supply the body; an over-secretion or a diminished supply of which impairs, as the case may be, the functions of the various organs through which they pass.

We will now concentrate our attention upon the

Functional Processes of Digestion,

which are as follows:—1st, prehension, or the grasping of food; 2d, mastication, or the chewing of food; 3d, insalivation, or the mixture of the food with saliva and other secretions of the mouth; 4th, deglutition, or the act by which substances are passed from the mouth into the stomach; 5th, rumination, a function peculiar to ruminating animals, by which they chew a second time the food they have swallowed (an analogous phenomenon is sometimes observed in man); 6th, chylification, or the formation of chyle during the digestive process; 7th, chymification, or the formation of chyme; 8th, defecation, or the act by which the excrement is expelled from the body; 9th, urination, a function the result of which is the expulsion of matters, principally solid but held in solution, which have become unsuitable for nutrition. Now the tongue of the ox must be considered the true prehensile organ; it is rough and studded with *papillæ*, which look backwards. The upper lip is short and thick, and the incisors cut the food pressed against the pad. This process being finished, mastication follows. The food is then passed into the stomach, which is divided into four compartments, namely, the rumen, paunch, or first stomach; the reticulum, or second stomach; the omasum, or third stomach; and the abomasus, the lowermost or fourth stomach. The rumen is the largest stomach in the abdominal space; it is situated at the left side, having on its left side the spleen attached. The reticulum lies in front of this organ, the omasum and abomasus being on the right.

Internally the first stomach presents a rough appearance. The second is the smallest of the four, and its internal walls have the appearance of the cells of bees. The third stomach is remarkable for its numerous folds internally, these resembling the leaves of a book, which originated its familiar designation—the many-plies. These folds are from 100 to 130 in number, and are possessed of small hooks for catching the food that has escaped mastication. The fourth stomach is next in size to the first, and possesses a villous coat internally, with large longitudinal ridges, which disappear at the pyloric orifice or extreme end. This orifice closes the entrance into the intestinal canal.

Rumination.

It is a wonderful provision how the animal can delay this process at pleasure, so completely is it under the control of the will. Now the fluid that the first stomach contains is not secreted in it, but when an animal drinks, a portion of the water passes into it for the purpose of softening the food, which is again returned to the mouth for remastication. Again, when an animal swallows a pellet or mass of food, there is a pause, during which the lungs become inflated with air, which acts on the diaphragm, or, as it is often called, the midriff. This is a large muscle stretched transversely between the thoracic and abdominal cavities, or, in other words, the partition which separates the bowels and lungs. When, therefore, the diaphragm contracts, its fibres become straight, the chest is enlarged, and the abdomen diminished; it then acts as an inspiratory muscle. It may also, however, diminish the capacity of the chest, and thus act as an expiratory muscle as well. This muscle plays an important part in sighing, yawning, crying, coughing, sneezing, vomiting, hiccoughing, laughing, and in the expulsion of the fæces, &c., in man.

Now rumination is always accompanied by digestion, and is very easily disturbed; so much so, that the raising of an ox or cow will suspend it for a time. Hence it will be perceived that when your animals are chewing their cud, digestion is going on in its own natural way; therefore it is an error to disturb the reclining animal during this process. The reason I draw attention to this fact is because I have seen cattle habitually roused while this act was going on, more especially during the winter evenings, when it is customary to inspect all the stock at eight or nine o'clock, when they are often made to stand up to see if they stretch themselves, this being satisfactory evidence that all is well. But let me also impress this upon you, that the best sign you possibly can witness of good health is the ox or cow in the act of chewing the cud; therefore I repeat that it is a mistake to disturb an animal during this vital process.

Digestion.

This comprehends the entire series of changes by which the curdy material is converted into blood; it is a function by means of which alimentary substances, when introduced into the digestive canal, undergo different alterations, whose object it is to convert them into two parts : the one a reparatory juice, destined to renew the perpetual waste occurring in the animal economy; the other, after being deprived of its nutritious properties, is rejected from the body.

While the food remains in the stomach, it is kept at a temperature of 100 degrees, and subjected to a slow motion by the *peristaltic* action of that organ. It is slowly dissolved, the solution taking place at its surface as it gradually rolls or is carried to the entrance of the bowels. Again, while it continues in the stomach, the mucous surface of that organ is changed into a bright red colour, otherwise this membrane is usually pale. We also find a number of points on the internal surface of the stomach which discharge a clear fluid. This fluid assists in dissolving the food, and is called gastric juice, having an acid character. We now find that the food has become converted into chyme. This accumulates at the extremity of the stomach, the orifice of which opens and allows it to escape into the small intestines, where the bile is formed. It then separates into chyle, passing slowly along those channels (the intestinal canals), owing to the bile adhering to the walls. It is there absorbed by the lacteals, and finally converted into blood. These, then, are the functional processes of digestion. Let us next consider the diseases that affect the ox and cow.

Definition of Disease.

Disease comprehends, first, pathogeny, the generation, production, and development of disease; secondly, pathology, the branch of medicine whose object is the knowledge of thè nature and science of disease. It has been defined as diseased physiology and physiology of disease. It is divided into general and special; the first considers diseases in common, the second the particular history of each. It is again subdivided into internal or external, or medical and surgical. Thirdly, pathogenetic, the origin of disease; fourthly, semiology, or the symptoms of disease; fifthly, prognosis, a judgment formed by which we estimate the future progress and termination of disease; sixthly, diagnosis, the discrimination of disease by physical signs; for example, it is by the aggregate and succession of symptoms that a disease is detected. Again, symptom at one time was generally used in the same sense as sign; but with many, perhaps most of the present day, the former signifies a functional or vital phenomenon of disease, while the latter is applied to that which is more directly physical; and hence the expressions functional or vital phenomena or symptoms, in contradistinction to the physical signs afforded by auscultation and percussion. Seventhly, hygiene, or the part of medicine whose object is the preservation of health and the prevention of disease;

eighth and lastly, therapeutics, which signifies, "I wait upon, I alleviate, I attend upon the sick," or that part of medicine the object of which is the treatment of disease.

A disease is said to be contagious when it communicates itself to another by direct contact; infectious when communicated by *virus* or foul air; contagious when it affects animals that have been located in the same place; epizootic when it attacks a number of animals at the same time without any apparent cause; enzootic, peculiar to a district, where it arises from a local cause, although that cause may remain unknown. Sporadic supervenes indifferently in every season and situation, from accidental causes, and independently of any epidemic or contagious influence. Again, in cattle the nervous system is not so well developed as it is in the horse, consequently they are liable to a low typhoid form. Again, a narrow ox is more subject to disease than a well-formed one.

Proceeding now to the diseases that affect the alimentary canal, we will first notice those of the mouth, beginning with

Glossitis, or Inflammation of the Tongue.

The causes that come into operation to produce this disease are often very obscure. It is frequently due to the animal picking up poisonous herbs, or by the incautious administration of medicines, such as ammonia or turpentine. The usual symptoms are increased flow of saliva, great fever, mouth open, tongue swollen and hanging out, excessive pain, which, however, diminishes as swelling increases; finally, the patient loses all power over it, and general disturbance of the system ensues. Of course a patient in this condition refuses all food.

The Terminations of Glossitis

are the formation of abscesses, which may be considered favourable, as they generally take place at the base of the tongue, and burst sometimes through the intermaxillary space, or the hollow situated between the lower jaws. Should induration occur, it is greatly to be dreaded; therefore the best course to adopt is to consign the animal to a butcher, if it is in condition at all, for it will lose flesh rapidly. When, however, it is only an abscess, the treatment is very simple: open it with the lance, foment, and keep the patient on soft, sloppy food, always remembering to wash the mouth well after each diet.

There is another termination of inflammation of the tongue that is much to be dreaded, and is known as

Gangrene,

and may be defined as follows, namely, deprivation of life, or partial death of an organ. Some writers distinguish and divide mortification into two stages, naming the first incipient mortification or gangrene. It is attended with a sudden diminution of feeling in the part affected, livid discoloration, and detachment of the cuticle, under which a turbid fluid is effused, with crepitation owing to the disengagement of air into the areolar texture. When the part has become quite black and incapable of all feeling, circulation, and life, it constitutes the second stage, and is called *sphacelus*.

Gangrene, however, is frequently used synonymously with mortification, local *asphyxia* being the term employed for that condition in which the parts are in a state of suspended animation, and consequently susceptible of resuscitation. Again, when the part is filled with fluid in the process of becoming putrified, the affection is called *humid gangrene;* while, on the other hand, when it is dry and shrivelled, it constitutes *dry gangrene* or *mummification*.

Causes.—Violent inflammation, injuries, contusions, burns, congelation, a ligature applied to a large arterial trunk, mechanical obstruction to the return of blood, or by some inappreciable internal cause. Treatment, both of external and internal gangrene, varies according to the causes which produce them. For example, gangrene arising from excessive inflammation is obviated by antiphlogistics, or remedies opposed to inflammation, and that originating from intense cold by cautiously restoring the circulation by friction, &c. Again, when the gangrene has become developed, the separation of the *eschars* must be encouraged by emollient applications if there be considerable reaction, or by tonics and stimulants if the reaction be insufficient; or, if decided upon, remove the dead part. In doing this you must exercise considerable care lest the operation proves fatal. When animals recover from this disease they are usually slow feeders; and when drinking, they bury their heads, if practicable, up to the eyes in the water.

Prolapsus Linguæ, or Glossocele,

or protrusion of the tongue from the mouth. This disease depends generally on an inflammatory swelling of the organ. At times, however, a *chronic glossocele*, or sort of *œdematous* engorgement, is met with, which proceeds to a great length and deforms the dental arch and lips. The inflammatory aspect of the disease must be combated by antiphlogistics. If of an *œdematous* nature, such as is sometimes caused by excessive salivation, the infiltrated fluid may be pressed back by the hand of the practitioner, to get the tongue behind the teeth, and it may be retained there by a piece of gauze being strapped over the mouth; but if the animal has control over it, let it alone: if, on the other hand, he has lost that power, it may be necessary to amputate; afterwards dress with the usual dressings.

Choking.

Every one conversant with the habits of the ox and cow must have encountered occasional cases of choking. To the experienced in such matters it may be regarded as superfluous to offer any instruction, but our observations may assist the uninitiated in saving the life of many a valuable animal. Now it must be observed that in the majority of cases prompt and immediate means are of the greatest importance; nor will it be necessary to occupy space with any description of the materials that may cause obstruction. Suffice it to say that the ordinary cause of choking is either turnips, potatoes, or cake. The symptoms are likewise more or less familiar to every one, and can rarely be mistaken, as they conclusively direct attention to the throat. But it must also be remembered that the gullet at its commencement and termination is considerably narrower than the centre; therefore there is this danger to be encountered: supposing you succeed by manipulation in forcing the obstruction from the constricted upper portion of the tube, in all probability its course will be arrested at the other end, just before it reaches the entrance into the stomach. In such a case you may be induced to remove the precautionary means that you had employed to prevent swelling, as the evidence guides you to suppose that all danger is over. But such is not so, as you may have the painful experience of witnessing the death of your animal. It will, therefore, be advisable to study the satisfactory symptoms in order to avert this undesirable termination. Now the best evidence that can be observed, and which clearly demonstrates that the gullet is free from obstruction, is the animal's ability to swallow; when this function is restored, anxiety may be laid aside. These symptoms are so patent that it is impossible to arrive at any other than a correct diagnosis as to the cause.

Treatment.—Aided by two reliable strong men, you need have no fear to insert your hand as far down the throat as possible, and remove the offending substance. If you find that this cannot be accomplished, and the swelling increases, your next step must be to gag the patient. For this purpose a round piece of wood about nine inches long and two inches in diameter, with a large hole in the middle and a small hole at each end for passing a cord through, will be found to answer admirably. Secure this gag in the mouth above the tongue, and allow it to remain until the swelling in the first stomach has entirely subsided. Should there be a danger of the animal going down, and, through the excessive swelling, the bowels begin to obtrude, you must without any further delay have recourse to the trocar and canula, remembering always to insert the trocar into the left side, about four inches from the protuberance of bone. I have known instances where, through ignorance, the animal was punctured on the *right* side, the party excusing himself by declaring that he was always taught to consider that the right side was the proper place for this operation. The result was death. With reference to the probang or rammer, you are justified in using it if you think that you can accomplish the feat with safety; but if you have any scruple, you will be much safer to resort to the trocar, which, after insertion, you withdraw, leaving the canula to allow the free exit of gases; in fact, the tube ought not to be removed until you have effected a passage in the bowels by a good aperient, composed of Epsom salts and treacle, one pound of the former to two pounds of the latter. And let no one induce you to administer any medicine, either in the solid or liquid state, while the throat is obstructed, for should you employ any agent for the purpose of softening the material that has effected a lodgment in the gullet, it is almost a foregone conclusion that immediate death will be the result. Some people open the poor animal's mouth and throw salt down the throat, in order to induce it to cough up the foreign body. The practice is to be condemned, for the results are unsatisfactory. Again, should it be necessary to cut into the gullet in order to remove the substance, the assistance of a professional man will be required.

Passing on now to the diseases proper, let us begin with one that is of frequent occurrence; one which, if not speedily arrested, often terminates fatally. It is called

Tympanitis, Hoven, or Distension of the First Stomach.

It is produced by the fermentation of food in this organ, and occurs most commonly in spring, when the grasses are luxurious and tempting; or when the animal is getting tares or fitches, more especially when they are wet with dew. Tympanitis may be either idiopathic or symptomatic, the former depending upon the exhalation of air from the decomposition of substances contained within the stomach, or from obstruction in the digestive tube. This form of the disease is not difficult to cure. But the symptomatic form is usually fatal. The symptoms are as follows:—Great distension of the stomach on the left side; if struck, it produces a hollow, drum-like sound; the nose is poked out; the breathing increases as the swelling increases; the hind-legs are drawn underneath the body; and if not speedily relieved, the animal drops down and dies from rupture of the stomach.

Treatment.—When the distension is great and no convenient remedy is at hand, insert the trocar into the stomach at once, and liberate the gases. If you have not a trocar in your possession, a sharp-pointed knife will do in a case of emergency.

Your next step must be to gag the mouth with the piece of wood already described in Choking. Allow this to remain until you have procured the proper remedies. These consist of ammonia, which, from its double action as an antacid and stimulant, is of special value, because it not only controls the nervous force, but it counteracts spasms,—the dose for cattle being from two to ten drachms, largely diluted with gruel; ether comes next, the dose of which is two to three ounces in water or gruel; alcohol next, and turpentine, when it is impossible to procure those other remedies. Exercise and friction must also be called into requisition, and a good dose of aperient medicine administered. When the physic has operated, remove the tube from the side, and as a rule the patient makes a satisfactory recovery. But, again, chronic tympanitis may follow as a sequel, and affect the animal in a variety of forms, which return at short intervals. It may be due to an error in feeding, indigestion, or organic disease of the internal coats of the stomach; or it may be owing to a distension of the walls of that organ and their inability to contract.

Treatment.—Administer a laxative, change entirely the diet, and follow up with tonics and sedatives. This disease rarely affects calves, but it is a malady that frequently attacks sheep, and is felt very severely when it does so.

Impaction of the First Stomach

occurs in both cattle and sheep, and is a much more serious disease than tympanitis. The symptoms are swelling in the region of the left flank and side; and if you press the stomach with your hand, you will find it very hard and unyielding, while it produces a dull-like sound when struck. The patient will be very often stupid from the commencement, and always evinces great irritation, which is accompanied by deep groans. The breathing will be greatly quickened owing to the walls of the stomach pressing against the diaphragm. This disorder also requires energetic treatment, therefore an active dose of medicine must be given, and on no account permit food to be partaken of. Should the bowels not be relieved within twelve hours, repeat the physic and follow up with stimulants. If, however, this course of treatment produces no beneficial results, then you must have recourse to the operation called rumenotomy—that is to say, you make a bold deep incision through the side and stomach, of such magnitude as will allow your hand to penetrate into the interior, when of course you remove from the stomach the offending cause. Having accomplished this, the next step is to carefully stitch up the stomach and side, which must first be well cleansed. Exercise particular caution with reference to diet, attend to the general comfort of the patient, keeping it as free from movement as possible.

The Second Stomach

generally becomes involved in any disease which affects the first. It is, however, rarely the seat of any important disease itself, but it seems to be the residence where foreign bodies accumulate when swallowed. The third stomach or many-plies is liable to a disease called

Fardel-Bound or Impaction.

It is simply a constipation of this organ, which may be involved in all diseases.

Symptoms. — These vary according to severity. Rumination ceases; the animal refuses all food, even of the most tempting description; the secretion of milk becomes arrested, with fever present; horns warm at the roots but cold at the tips: towards the third day the animal commences to grunt in a very characteristic, peculiar manner, and so closely does this grunt resemble that of pleuro-pneumonia, that it has often been confounded with the latter disease. After death the stomach is found to be enormously distended with hard, dry, indigestible food situated between the leaves of the organ. So hard indeed has this impacted material become, that you can rub it down between your finger and thumb.

Treatment.—It is important to administer a very powerful purgative—in fact, you can scarcely give too strong a dose ; follow up with stimulants, and apply hot fomentations to the right side. If stupor or frenzy takes place, little or no hope can be entertained. If, however, the patient still remains conscious, and the medicine you administered at first inactive, say after eighteen or twenty hours, give the following draught :—Three-quarters of a pound each of Epsom and common table salts, and, when obstinate, twenty croton beans, with one drachm of calomel, given in four or five quart bottles of gruel. Along with stimulants, such as ammonia, ale, ether, or spirits, injections may be given, but I have no faith in their reaching the seat of disease ; they only overload the bowels without effecting any serviceable object.

The third stomach is also liable to inflammation, the symptoms of which are somewhat analogous to fardel-bound, with this addition, that there is a peculiar twitching of the muscles of the head and neck, accompanied with a staggering gait and tucked-up belly.

Treatment.—Hot fomentations, linseed-oil internally, with opium, and nitre in the water given to drink.

The fourth stomach is liable to many diseases

that appertain to the others, the most common of which is indigestion and functional derangement, thought to be caused by undue activity, but often due to the kind of food.

Symptoms.—The coat becomes coarse and staring, appetite capricious; the animal licks the wall or any cold substance with its tongue; if in a cow, the milk is poor and scanty, and frequently diarrhœa ensues.

Treatment.—Give an alkaline combined with an aromatic and stimulant, and food in small quantities, with rock salt placed in a trough within the animal's reach; this must be followed up with gentle exercise and plenty of pure fresh air.

The fourth stomach is also liable to true inflammation, but this is fortunately of rare occurrence. The most frequent cause is due to the animal eating some poisonous substance, such as the leaves of the ordinary yew-tree, &c. The symptoms are great pain and frequent attempts to vomit; the animal appears languid and sleepy; frequently attempts to pass fæces; whilst after death intense inflammation of the stomach is evidenced.

Treatment.—Get rid of the poison or neutralise it; but first examine into the circumstances of the case to enable you to know what kind of neutralising agent will be required; also give a purgative, with opium and mild stimulants.

Inflammation.

This is, as the term signifies, a setting on fire, and is so alarming, that whenever the expression escapes the speaker's lips, the announcement is received by every one conversant with the ailments of the lower animals with the utmost concern and anxiety.

Bleeding, the pet remedy with many, is it really worthy of consideration ? This being a question of considerable importance in the treatment of inflammation, we will dispose of it first.

In discussing this blood-letting remedy, many suppose, assert, and maintain that by its adoption you diminish the inflammatory process going on in any organ or region of the body. Such an idea is entirely fallacious, and a little examination into the character of blood, and how it acts in an inflamed organ or part, will clearly demonstrate its absurdity; for where we find inflammation, there the circulation becomes arrested, and stagnation is the result.

How then is this stoppage to be got rid of ? Certainly not by bleeding, since the blood has become coagulated in the part, and therefore can no longer flow. So if recourse is had to this remedy, you diminish the strength of the patient, impair its vitality, increase exhaustion, and hasten death, because you have removed the principal power of resistance.

Take a practical analogy. Supposing you have a stopped drain to contend with, you are aware that water is not the obstruction, but that there is some material which has effected a lodgment, owing to which the water is directed out of its usual channel. In such a case you would consider it extreme folly to open the drain at a distance of seven or eight feet from the obstructing material, therefore you have your opening made in the immediate vicinity of the stoppage in order to reach the cause, which, once reached and removed, the water resumes its course uninterruptedly. This is exactly the position with bleeding. The blood is not the obstruction or the cause of inflammation, but it is the irritant that has effected a residence in the part; hence the inflammation as a result of this irritant. Remove this irritant, then, as you would remove the obstructive material from the drain; and when you accomplish this, the bad effects will cease, and the inflammatory process will be arrested.

We will now proceed to the definition of inflammation given by some of our leading authorities. Dr. Hunter says:—" Inflammation is due to an increased action of vessels, observing at the same time that dilatation of the vessels was as much an evidence of power as the contraction." And again he says:— " Such is inflammation, blood much altered, stagnant, or tending to stagnation; capillaries over-distended, the coats of which are spongy, soft, and lacerable; copious exudation of liquor sanguinis; extravasation of blood by lesion of capillary coats; absorption in abeyance; nutrition and function perverted; structure changed; texture softened and enlarged; suppuration in progress with part of texture breaking up; nothing healthy or consistent with local health; all essentially diseased." Professor Syme says:—"It is a peculiar perverted action of the capillary system, attended by pain, heat, redness, and swelling." Dr. Alison says:— "It is a peculiar perversion of nutrition or of secretion." The cause then of this *stasis* or stagnation is an irritant, which irritation must be looked upon as one of three processes : first, nutritive; second, functonal; third, formative.

Having now this irritant as the exciting cause, if the part is vascular—for inflammation cannot exist in a part containing no blood-vessels, but exists in the parts immediately surrounding it— the nutrition becomes perverted, then congestion of the parts takes place, while the capillaries first contract, then dilate, and the blood meantime, flowing slowly, becomes irregular and oscillates, until complete stagnation occurs. At this period the vessels become greatly distended, the red globules of the blood grow adhesive and stick to the walls of the vessels, while they also adhere one to the other.

Again, in some cases the vessels present dilatations of their whole circumference at certain parts of their course, due to the thin parts of the wall bulging out from the accumulated pressure of blood within.

The next process is the extravasation of serum (namely, the watery portion of the blood) into the surrounding tissues. This also takes place in health; but in inflammation the quantity exuded or given off is in greater abundance than is required, and has to be absorbed by the cells of the surrounding tissue, thereby producing enlargement of the parts.

Again, the blood may extravasate from rupture of the vessel's coats. Should this occur, sudden obstacles spring up, which suspend the life of the parts for a time, and, if very acute, may destroy it altogether.

Some writers assert that constriction of the vessels never takes place prior to the dilatation. If you irritate a part with weak vinegar, the constriction takes place very slowly; but when you apply a strong acid, the constriction is so rapid that it passes into the dilated condition almost at once. The dilatation, then, is of a passive nature, and arises from the walls being unable to resist the pressure of the blood, as they are weakened and debilitated.

Stasis, or complete stagnation, then, is due to the increased vitality of the tissues themselves, which draw the blood towards them like a loadstone attracting iron to itself.

Having now directed your attention to this indisputable fact, pointing out the origin of inflammation, and how an irritant exerts its power over the circulation until it has finally arrested the flow of blood, you will perceive that blood-letting, if resorted to generally, must have a pernicious effect upon the subject, and ought, in the name of justice and sympathy, to be for ever abandoned.

In considering another remedy intimately allied with blood-letting for the treatment of inflammation, it will be necessary, in the first place, to direct your attention to an important element in the blood, known as fibrin.

Fibrin, although occupying a minor position as to quantity, is nevertheless one of the most essential constituents of the circulating fluid. It has something like a percentage of four to five, but may vary occasionally. It is through this fibrin that the wounds of vessels heal up, and if it were not for this material a mere scratch would have a fatal issue. In infants, for example, when a vessel is cut or wounded, it is a matter of extreme difficulty to arrest the flow of blood: this is due to a want of fibrin.

Again, in black-quarter, or black-leg, as it is sometimes called, the disease occurs merely owing to a deficiency of this fibrinous element in the blood.

Let us consider the treatment, or rather the prevention, of this fatal disease. It is by means of counter-irritation that you can secure success, or by the insertion of a seton into the dewlap, which is the most rapid way of combating the attack when it appears amongst a herd of cattle. By this means fibrin is formed in the parts, and taken up by the absorbents, and then carried into the blood. That being satisfactorily explained in the effectual prevention of black-leg, surely it must be accepted as unmistakable evidence that counter-irritation is opposed to the successful treatment of inflammation, as it increases the fibrin enormously; hence increased coagulation of the blood in an inflamed part is the inevitable result, since it accelerates stagnation, thus rendering it impossible for the blood to flow. Blistering, then, so often resorted to in the treatment of inflammation, is a direct manufacturer of fibrin; and knowing the part this constituent plays during inflammation, I have no hesitation in denouncing it as bad treatment for the disease under discussion.

The only conclusion, therefore, that I can arrive at with safety is, that soothing remedies are the only successful and legitimate ones to be employed; and that counter-irritants, being pathologically against recovery, are consequently accompanied with danger to vital parts.

We will now consider the local symptoms of inflammation, which are as follows:—1st, Redness; 2d, Heat; 3d, Pain; 4th, Swelling; 5th, Loss of Function.

First, then, Redness in the lower animals cannot be well observed, and is only seen upon the white spots and the visible mucous membrane. It is caused by the engorged state of the capillaries and the blood-globules being dissolved, thus tinging the tissues with hæmatin, which is the colouring matter of the blood. The redness is deepest in the centre, and gradually pales off toward the circumference of the inflamed parts; but if caused by extravasation, it will not be removed by pressure (as in true inflammation), therefore the aspect of redness differs according to various circumstances. If the inflamed vessels be uniformly distended, they will be of a uniform deep blush; and if observed in the mouth, they will appear as folds of red velvet.

After stagnation has become complete, the tissues are stained by this extravasated colouring matter of the blood, hæmatin; and when a *post-mortem* examination is made, if the subject has lain upon its back, the muscles of the back will be found completely congested and red. This, however, is owing to the force of gravity drawing the blood to the lowest parts of the patient; and the same appearances will always present themselves, no matter in what position the subject is lying, provided it has lain long enough. When such takes place after death, it is termed hypostatic redness.

The presence or absence of redness is not of itself a proof of inflammation; for in inflammation of the cornea, one of the membranes of the eye, or articular cartilage, or arachnoid membrane, there is no redness, but the parts are opaque or white.

Heat.—The temperature of the inflamed part seems higher both to the observer and patient, but the increase of heat is not so decided as one would imagine. Dr. Hunter proved that the temperature is only one degree higher than the other parts. The greatest amount of heat in an inflamed part is where it is seated far distant from the centre of circulation, and in parts where the heat of the blood is several degrees lower than that of the heart; therefore the sense of heat that the patient endures must be due to the increased sensibility of the part, combined with the nervous functions.

Experiments have shown that the blood going to an inflamed part is less warm than the part itself, and that venous blood returning from an inflamed part is warmer than that returning from other parts. And again, in inflammation of a region near the centre of circulation, instead of the temperature of the blood being increased, it is actually diminished.

Pain.—The pain of inflammation varies much in degree and duration, according to its cause, intensity, and seat.

In loose structures the pain is dull compared to dense, strong, fibrous tissues. The pain of open joints, laminitis, &c., is of the most acute nature;

and in pleurisy,—the pain being of a sharp, darting description,—is often mistaken for colic.

In acute peritonitis (the covering membrane of the bowels), the pain is so agonising that the animal is terrified to move a limb, therefore it does not show much suffering.

Again, the pain of an inflamed mucous membrane does not always amount to acute pain, therefore its presence or absence does not always indicate inflammation; and the sudden cessation of pain in violent inflammation is much to be dreaded, as it unmistakably shows that the vitality of the part has been destroyed, or, in other words, gangrene has set in.

Again, the situation of pain is not always the seat of inflammation, as in inflammation of the liver the pain is felt in the off shoulder, and the animal will go lame on that limb. This is termed "reflex pain."

In acute heart-disease the hind-legs are partially paralysed; this is called "sympathetic pain."

Cause of Pain.—Some writers ascribe pain to the pressure on the nerves of the part arising from exudation, while others maintain that the vessels of the part become slightly elongated and stretched by each impulse of the heart. I am assured, however, that it is owing to the actual germinal matters becoming greatly increased in the parts, as witnessed by the lines.

Swelling occurs independent of inflammation; and, according to some authorities, this symptom first depends upon the congested blood-vessels, with subsequent exudation and engorgement. But it depends upon the local production of lymph by the tissues on which it is found. When swelling occurs upon an external inflamed part, it may be looked upon as a favourable symptom, for exudation has taken place. But when swelling occurs upon any organ essential to life, such as the lungs, or even the throat, it may very soon terminate fatally.

Swelling, again, is not always characteristic of inflammation. For example, purpuræ hæmorrhagaica, scarlatina, &c., are diseases in which we have enormous swellings, yet they are not inflammatory ones.

Loss of Function, or impairment or perversion of the functions. In the first stage of inflammation, function may be increased, as in the first stages of phrenitis; but in the first stages of inflammation of the cornea the function is entirely or nearly suspended. In inflammation of the muscles their function is destroyed, while their sensibility is greatly increased.

The Terminations of Inflammation

are—1st, effusion of serum; 2d, exudation of coagulable lymph; 3d, suppuration; 4th, ulceration; 5th, gangrene; and 6th, resolution, which is said to occur when the parts resume their natural function.

Take, then, the first termination, which is effusion; this differs from exudation of lymph owing to the fact that it occurs in the loose areolar tissue, and partakes of the general constituents of serum. Serous effusion may result from mechanical congestion; and in such cases the fluid is clear, containing very little fibrin.

Now there are two essential characteristics of inflammatory effusion : 1st, It tends to contain ingredients in greater proportion than they exist in blood, namely, chlorates, phosphates, albuminates; 2d, They contain organic forms, and these forms find in this exudation a suitable situation for their growth.

In pneumonia, or inflammation of the lungs, in the human being, when the chlorate of soda is absent from the urine, it is an evidence that inflammation is going on as rapidly as ever; but as soon as it appears, we are justified in predicting a favourable termination.

Suppuration. — The formation of pus occurs in three different ways : 1st, circumscribed; 2d, diffused; 3d, superficial. In the first stage, the cells of the areolar tissue are charged with lymph, becoming enlarged, and for some time multiplying excessively. This is soon followed by a division of the cells themselves; and round about the inflamed part, where there were only single cells, pairs are now seen, and from them the new connective tissue is formed. Then, again, in the interior of this growth, where the cells were early filled, numberless little cells now appear, which at first preserve the form of the previous cellular tissue; and as these little cells extend in numbers and growth, the surrounding tissue liquefies, and pus is formed. A vital change has therefore taken place in the germs of the tissue, the whole process being effected in the cells themselves.

Healthy pus is a smooth, viscid, white or creamy-looking substance, having no odour and possessing an alkaline reaction. It is composed of two parts, cells and liquor puræ. When pus is formed near a bone or in the foot, it usually has a fetid smell, due to the death of the bone and the evolution of sulphuretted hydrogen. Pus consists of the following kinds: "laudable," or healthy; "ichorous," thin and watery; "sanious," mixed with blood.

2d, *Diffused.*—We find examples of this in the purulent effusions of a glandered horse; for there is no pointing, as the pus gravitates to the most depending parts.

3d, *Superficial Suppuration*, met with in the mucous membranes and skin. All mucous membranes, with only a single layer of epithelium, are much less adapted to the formation of pus. Again, the intestinal mucous membrane scarcely ever produces pus without ulceration; but all mucous membranes can secrete pus without ulceration, and that through a change in their epithelial scales.

Ulceration.—This takes place in the living tissue surrounding the dead. A groove is formed in the red line by the absorption of the living tissue; this line deepens, and the pus formed burrows in and removes the slough, below which a healthy granulating surface is exposed.

Mortification consists of two kinds—complete and incomplete.

In the soft structure the complete is termed sphacelus, the incomplete gangrene. When it exists in the blood it is termed necræmia. Again, when the dead tissue is visible, it is termed a "slough," and the process by which it is removed "sloughing."

Degeneration may be distinguished from mortification, as in it the fat does not become decomposed, and pus is not formed to carry it off by separation from the healthy part.

Mortification may be either wet or dry. It is wet or moist when the blood exudes and then separates into its various constituents. Dry mortification is rarely seen, but has been found to follow on the use of ergot of rye.

Necræmia, or death of the blood, is seen in splenic apoplexy, quarter-ill, and the last stages of rinderpest. In those diseases there are large patches of dead and decomposed blood absorbed by the tissues, causing swelling, which crepitates on pressure.

Mortification may arise, without inflammation, from a stoppage of blood to the part, or it may be brought about by the vessels being absorbed or destroyed by ulceration. When mortification ceases to spread, a red line is observed around its circumference, separating the dead from the living parts, which testifies that a process has been established for the removal of the dead tissue. The healthy tissue in the meantime becomes consolidated; the mouths of the blood-vessels are sealed up; there is no hæmorrhage, and the virus from the dead portion cannot be taken up by these healthy blood-vessels.

Again, mortification may take place from actual contact with other parts, as witnessed in death from enteritis, where the bowel in its course comes in contact with any portion not already mortified.

Symptoms of inflammation are of two kinds—local and constitutional. Constitutional symptoms are indicative of sympathetic or inflammatory fever. These are of the greatest importance, signifying the nature of the disease when internally seated. The most prominent symptoms are the rigors, or shivering fits that usher in the disease. These rigors are followed by an increased heat of the skin; the pulse is firm and hard, accompanied by more or less disturbance of the natural functions of the animal's body. The rigors are often very severe, while occasionally they may amount only to mere chilliness. They are, however, important, as they mark the commencement of the disease or fever. Again, rigors oftener attend spontaneous inflammation than that caused by an irritant. Some animals with weak constitutions are peculiarly liable to rigors.

Fever, then, is the effect of inflammation, and during the inflammatory process one of the most important changes that occur in the blood is the increase of fibrin, which encourages coagulation very rapidly at the inflamed parts.

Treatment.—If an animal is suffering from an injury of any kind, the first duty incumbent upon us is to prevent inflammation by removing the cause. The local remedies must be soothing, with complete repose strictly enjoined. If these preliminary steps be neglected or imperfectly performed, the most energetic remedies may be employed, but they will avail little, as the disease will then have got a firm hold. For instance, you may have a prick of the foot, and the source of the injury remain unnoticed. You may bleed, purge, and do everything, but unless you remove the cause your efforts are in vain.

The old antiphlogistic theory led practitioners to bleed for everything, and that to an enormous extent. But having already given you my opinion upon the matter, it is not necessary here to recur to the subject again. Suffice it to say, once for all, that the operation of bleeding is opposed to all sound theory.

The next step, then, to be taken is a purgative, as

it frees the intestinal canal from all irritating matter; for this purpose Epsom salts and treacle are the best. Purgatives, however, must be cautiously administered; for if we have a case of thoracic inflammation—that is, inflammation of the organs that are contained within the cavity of the chest—they must not be administered; but with stomach, brain, liver, and bowel affections, accompanied with general derangement, it is impossible to over-estimate their value.

The next salutary remedy that possesses extraordinary soothing power, that subdues pain, allays nervous irritability, and is invaluable when given in a watery solution, is opium. Aconite comes next, but is most useful in inflammation accompanied by excitement rather than pain. It improves the tone and diminishes the frequency of the pulse; and I have witnessed the most encouraging evidence of its successful action.

Belladonna is another useful agent, but it is principally beneficial in allaying irritation attending sore-throat.

Amongst the neutral remedies, potassa nitras possesses the power of dissolving the fibrin in the blood, and prevents the formation of it by the tissues; while it increases the secretion of urine, and assists particularly the expulsion by this channel of the products derived from the destruction of the albuminous materials of the body. It should always be given in large quantities of cold water, as it is then readily assimilated by the blood; but if given in a concentrated form in the animal's food, it abstracts water from the blood, thus rendering it thick, which is not desirable.

Grass Staggers.

This kind of disease is of frequent occurrence during summer, but it will appear at any season, provided the animals are exposed to the exciting cause, which is hard, dry, indigestible food. It is worst when the seed is on the different grasses, while it is often met with in cows that are fed on tares. Indeed, so closely connected is this disease with this kind of herbage, that the two stand in relation to each other as positive cause and effect. The symptoms, to the uninitiated, may point in the direction of the brain, and if treated accordingly, it will be without success.

Symptoms.—These appear gradually. The animal looks dull and listless, and cannot use the hind-legs properly, accompanied by a staggering sort of gait. Sometimes these symptoms disappear, and the animal will seem in apparent health for two or three days; however, the disease will very likely soon manifest itself again by drowsiness and hanging head, with irregular torpidity of the bowels. The animal takes a mouthful of food, quids it, and then lets it drop along with a quantity of saliva. This state may continue for other two or three days, sometimes a week, and even a fortnight, when it gets gradually worse. The animal now pokes the nose into a corner, resting the lower jaw upon any convenient place. Shortly after this it falls on one side, throws back the head towards the side, and frequently goes into a convulsive fit. These fits occur at short intervals, when death soon ends the struggle.

Post-mortem Appearances.—Fæces hard and dry, with impaction of the third stomach, and sometimes the first stomach. Patches of inflammation will be also found in the intestinal canal, often accompanied by congestion of the lungs; this, however, is not due to the disease, but to nervous prostration. The vessels about the brain and spinal chord are also tinged with dark blood, which explains the general dulness of the patient during life. Derangement, then, of the stomach and intestines is the primary cause of the brain symptoms. As these organs are plentifully supplied with nerves from the brain and spinal cord, impressions are conveyed through this nervous communication to the nerve centres; hence the feeling of oppression, which is succeeded by the unsteady gait.

Treatment.—The first object must be to get the stomach and bowels unloaded; this is accomplished by administering a strong purgative, followed up with stimulants. Some authors recommend setons and blisters to the top of the head; but for the reasons already adduced, I cannot advise their application. Besides, I hold they are entirely uncalled for, seeing that the disease has its origin in the stomach; therefore the cause must be removed. When this is successfully accomplished, little more will be required but to exercise moderation in feeding in future, and a total change of diet.

Description of the Intestines.

The small intestines are divided into three portions; namely, the *duodenum, jejunum,* and *ileum.* The duodenum is the first part of the intestinal canal, commencing at the pyloric orifice of the stomach, and terminating in the jejunum. In the duodenum chylification takes place after the admixture of the biliary and pancreatic fluids with the chyme. The jejunum is the part of the small intestines comprised between the duodenum and ileum. The ileum comes next, and completes the series of small bowels.

The large intestines are likewise divided into three portions; namely, the *cæcum, colon,* and *rectum.* The cæcum, or blind gut—so called from its being open at one end only—is that portion of the intestinal canal which is seated between the termination of the ileum and commencement of the colon, the ileo-cæcal valve shutting off all communication between them. The colon is that portion of the large intestines which extends from the cæcum to the rectum;

while the rectum is the third and last portion of the great intestines. This organ receives the fæcal matters as they pass from the colon, and serves as a reservoir for this material.

Constipation

is a state of the bowels in which the evacuations do not take place as frequently as usual, or are inordinately hard and expelled with great difficulty. It may be due to diminished action of the muscular coat of the intestines, or to diminished secretion from the mucous membrane, or to both, but it is frequently due to impaction of the third stomach.

Treatment.—Cathartic medicines will usually remove it; after which, its exciting and predisposing causes must be inquired into and removed, to render cure permanent.

Diarrhœa

is a disease characterised by frequent liquid alvine evacuations, and is generally a result of inflammation or irritation of the mucous membrane of the intestines. It is also often caused by errors in feeding—the use of unwholesome food, given in large quantities. This disease is frequently an effort of nature to get rid of the irritating matters that become lodged in the intestines. Intestinal worms are another cause, and young grass; also nervous excitement and disorders of the blood, &c.

Symptoms. — Frequent evacuations; considerable straining; appetite not much impaired; seldom pain or fever, and pulse not much affected.

Treatment.—Diarrhœa requires different remedies according to its nature. If caused, as it often is, by improper matters in the intestinal canal, these must be got rid of by a gentle purge, such as linseed-oil and carbonate of soda. If the discharges seem to be kept up by irritability of the intestines, the astringent plan must be adopted, combined with tonics and aromatics. The following will be found useful: —Dilute sulphuric acid, one drachm, tincture of opium, one ounce, given in starch or gruel, twice a day; or, catechu, half an ounce, with gentian or ginger, two or three times a day, in warm sweet ale, accompanied with entire change of food.

White Scour in Calves, Diarrhœa.

The cause of this ailment is generally traceable to the food, which of course must be changed; then administer linseed or castor oil, or Epsom salts and treacle, with a stimulant, such as spirits of ether or alcohol. When the bowels are cleaned out, give a switched egg and a little port-wine and ginger mixed, attending at the same time to the general comfort of the patient.

Dyspepsia in Calves

is a state of the stomach in which its functions are disturbed without the presence of other diseases. If other diseases are present, they are but of minor importance.

The Symptoms are various. Those affecting the stomach are,—loss of appetite; animal dull and listless; hide-bound, and pain on pressure at the right side of the belly. The sympathetic affections are of the most diversified character; but the disease, being generally of a functional nature, is devoid of danger. However, it may arise from disease of the stomach itself, when it becomes more serious. It is usually produced by irregularity in feeding, or in the quantity or quality of the food. It is often connected with an inflammatory or sub-inflammatory condition of the mucous lining of the stomach. Dyspepsia is also often attended with too great a secretion of the gastric acids; and in many cases they would appear to be too small in quantity, so as to constitute alkaline or neutral indigestion.

Treatment.—Purgative, with change of diet.

Dysentery, or Bloody Flux,

is an inflammatory condition of the mucous membrane of the intestines, the chief symptoms of which are as follows:—Fever, more or less inflammatory; frequent mucous or bloody evacuations; appetite capricious; rumination ceases; lifting of the flanks; animal stands with its head down, tail erect; dark-red urine; abdominal pain varies considerably, accompanied with distension of the first stomach, great thirst, emaciation, eruptions on the mouth, in some cases abscesses, and in others ulceration.

Treatment is very uncertain. Give mild laxatives, such as linseed and castor oil, and adopt the same course as for diarrhœa.

Colic.

This disease only occurs in the ox and cow in the spasmodic form. The flatulent form of colic is seen in tympanitis. It is, however, very rare in cattle, but it arises from the same cause that produces it in the horse; that is, by indigestion, causing muscular contraction of the coats of the intestines. The symptoms are more sudden and violent than in the horse : great restlessness, stamping the ground with the feet, shifting from one leg to another, constipation, and frequently tympanitis.

Treatment.—An active aperient is generally all that is required, when the disease will either terminate in recovery or

Enteritis, or Inflammation of the Bowels.

The essential symptoms of this disease are violent abdominal pain, which is increased on pressure, with inflammatory fever; the muzzle is hot and dry; pulse quick and strong; lifting of the flanks; urine scanty and high-coloured; shifting of the feet, kicking the belly, grinding the teeth, flow of saliva from the mouth; sometimes constipation, at other times slimy evacuations; extremities cold; pulse becomes quicker and feebler, the animal dying totally exhausted. Causes: eating poisonous plants, wet pastures, bad food or water, over-driving, &c. Enteritis may affect both the peritoneal and the mucous coats of the intestines, the former of which covers, while the latter lines the bowels; and in violent cases all the coats may be implicated. But the structure of the mucous and peritoneal coats is different. So are their functions in health and disease. The inflammation of the serous coat resembles that of the cellular membrane; the inflammation of the mucous coat that of the skin. The former is usually, therefore, of a more active character. Again, inflammation of the mucous coat is generally attended with diarrhœa, and its pathology is identical with that of dysentery.

Inflammation of the peritoneal coat is, on the other hand, generally attended with constipation.

Treatment.—Hot fomentations carefully and persistently applied to the abdomen. Tincture of opium in two-ounce doses every three hours; linseed-oil or Epsom salts and treacle as a purge, encouraging the animal to drink tepid water with nitre dissolved in it.

Peritonitis.

Enteritis of the peritoneal coat—for such literally is the meaning of the word—requires the most active remedies. However, it is a rare disease amongst cattle, but may occur as a sequel to castration, or from violence inflicted upon an animal. It is generally ushered in by a shivering fit; the pulse will be hard and wiry, accompanied with great restlessness, shifting of the feet, straining, grinding of the teeth, great fever, and violent pain.

Treatment.—The same remedies that are employed for enteritis, with a plentiful supply of hot water fomentations to the abdomen.

Dropsy, or Ascites,

may occur as a sequel to the former disease. It is an accumulation of fluid in the abdomen, which may be the result of a weakening of the capillary vessels, these allowing the watery portion of the blood to exude through their walls. The abdomen becomes of an enormous size; there is no pain evinced upon pressure, but the breathing and pulse are hurried. It is rarely a primary disease, but is always dangerous, and but little susceptible of cure. The treatment to adopt is diuretics, stimulants, and, if no benefit can be derived from these, paracentesis, or tapping, must be had recourse to. However, it can only be regarded as a palliative. When this operation is performed, you make an incision in the skin six or eight inches from the anterior part of the udder, and about one inch from the linea alba—that is, the line that runs directly along the middle of the abdomen. You then insert the trocar and canula, when the fluid is easily removed. You must now give good nourishing food, with stimulants and tonics.

Prolapsus Ani and Uteri.

This occurs in all domestic animals, and is a protrusion of the bowel and womb. The causes are violent straining or intestinal worms, which often produce great irritation; hence the frequent attempts to get rid of them. It is sometimes not a very easy task to return either of these organs, but the following method will greatly facilitate the operation:—You must elevate the hind-quarters as high as you possibly can, and well wash the organs that are to be returned with warm water. It may be also necessary to wash with a dilute solution of opium and carbolic acid; then return very carefully. Afterwards you must either apply a truss or close the external opening by means of a suture. Give a dose of opium, say two ounces, or chloral, two ounces, in order to control or prevent straining. Either of these agents will suit the purpose admirably, keeping the animal quiet and comfortable, and allowing nothing but soft, easily digestible food in moderate quantity.

DISEASES OF THE ACCESSORY ORGANS OF DIGESTION.

Hepatitis, or Inflammation of the Liver.

The liver is a highly organised gland, situated within the abdominal cavity behind the diaphragm. It is the largest secreting gland in the body. It is unsymmetrical, very heavy, and of a brownish-red colour; it is surrounded by a serous or peritoneal covering. The blood-vessels in the liver are very numerous. The hepatic artery and vena porta furnish it with the blood necessary for its nutrition and the secretion of bile; the hepatic veins convey away the blood which has served those purposes. The lymphatic vessels are also very numerous, some being superficial, others deeply seated. The nerves are also very plentiful, and proceed from the pneumogastric, diaphragmatic, and the hepatic plexuses.

The intricate structure of the liver has been well studied. When cut, it presents a porous appearance, owing to the division of a multitude of small vessels; when torn, it seems formed of granulations, the structure of which has given rise to many hypotheses. In these granulations are contained the radicles of the excretory ducts of the bile, the union of which constitutes the hepatic duct. The internal structure of the liver consists of a number of lobules composed of *intralobular* or *hepatic* veins, which convey the blood back that has been used in the secretion of bile. The *interlobular* plexus of veins is formed by branches of the vena porta, which contain both the blood of the vena porta and of the hepatic artery, both of which are considered to furnish the pabulum of the biliary secretion. The biliary ducts form likewise an *interlobular* plexus, having an arrangement similar to that of the interlobular veins.

The liver is perhaps the only organ which, independently of the red blood carried to it by the hepatic artery, receives black blood by the vena porta, the general opinion being that the blood of the vena porta furnishes the bile, whilst the hepatic artery affords blood for the nutrition of the organ itself. It is probable, however, that bile is secreted from the blood of the latter vessel. Besides bile, the liver forms sugar, and is the great assimilating organ. It also produces glycogen or animal starch, which is readily converted into sugar. Hepatitis or inflammation of the liver may be seated either in the peritoneal covering or in the substance of the liver. It may be also either acute or chronic.

Acute inflammation occurs rarely in the ox, but it may be brought on by the animal being highly fed and having no exercise, or a sudden change from bad to good food, which causes a great secretion of bile; as a result of this, the gland becomes engorged with blood, and inflammation is set up.

Symptoms.—The patient is dull and listless, but

indicates no severe pain; the skin is rough and itchy; the mucous membranes of a reddish-yellow colour; tongue foul; rumination arrested; small quantities of fæces are evacuated: sometimes these are dark and glossy, at other times they are of a whitish, clay-looking colour, having a fetid smell. Should the peritoneal covering become implicated, the febrile symptoms are very severe: dropsy is the result, with great emaciation and death.

Treatment.—It is of the utmost importance to relieve the bowels as soon as possible; for this purpose give a good saline purge with one drachm of calomel; when this has operated, it will relieve the blood-vessels of the liver. Apply plenty of hot water to the right side over the region of the organ, and allow as much pure water, with nitre dissolved in it, as the patient can drink: restrict the diet, and prevent food of a stimulating nature being given.

Chronic Hepatitis.

The primary symptoms of this disease are not easily defined, but the animal will be found dull, listless, hide-bound; appetite lost or capricious, bowels constipated; fæces that may be passed are hard, dark, or clay-coloured, while rumination is suspended. Chronic hepatitis is generally far advanced before the services of a professional man are requested.

Treatment.—Saline purge with calomel, frequently

repeated, and an active blister over the region of the liver, may exercise a wholesome influence. The *post-mortem* appearances reveal the organ as large, soft, and friable, and frequently attached to the surrounding parts.

Icterus, Jaundice, or Yellows.

This disease generally follows debilitating affections, but it may also occur as an idiopathic from various causes. In fact, anything that may obstruct, directly or indirectly, the course of the bile, so that it is taken into the mass of blood, produces the yellowness of the skin and eyes. The bile being separated by the kidneys causes yellowness of the urine, and its being prevented from reaching the intestines occasions pale, clay-coloured fæces. The disease, however, is more common to the human subject than to our patients; the reason being that cattle are select in their beverages, and don't indulge in anything stronger than water, which exercises no deleterious or pernicious effect upon this important organ, the liver. The prognosis in ordinary cases is very satisfactory, but when it is complicated with hepatic disease, it becomes unfavourable. The treatment is simple. Were it admissible to give an emetic, that would often be all that is required; but, for the best of reasons, we cannot induce the ox or cow to vomit as readily as man. We have therefore to rely upon an active purge, so as to encourage the return of bile to its ordinary channels. Give also light, easily digested tonics and soothing diet, always remembering to keep the bowels open.

Biliary Calculi, or Gall-Stones.

Calculi are concretions which may form in any part of the animal body, but are most frequently found in the organs which act as reservoirs, and in the excretory canals. They are met with in the tonsils, joints, biliary ducts, digestive passages, lachrymal ducts, mammæ, pancreas, lungs, salivary, spermatic, and urinary passages, and in the womb. The causes which give rise to them are obscure.

Those that occur in reservoirs or ducts are supposed to be owing to the deposition of the substances which compose them from the fluid as it passes along the duct, and those which occur in the substance of an organ are regarded as the product of some nutritive irritation. Their general effect is to irritate, as extraneous bodies, the parts with which they are in contact, and to produce retention of the fluid by which they have been formed. The symptoms differ according to the sensibility of the organ and the importance of the particular secretion whose discharge they impede. Their solution is usually impracticable; spontaneous expulsion or extraction is the only way of getting rid of them.

Biliary calculi appear to contain all the materials

of the bile, and seem to be nothing more than that secretion thickened. They are most frequently found in the gall-bladder, at other times in the substance of the liver, and when quiescent they often occasion no uneasiness. At other times, however, they cause violent inflammation, with sometimes rupture and fatal effusion into the peritoneum, the passage of a gall-stone being extremely painful.

Treatment of no avail.

Hypertrophy, or Chronic Enlargement of the Liver.

Owing to nutrition being performed with great activity, the liver becomes enormously enlarged. The *symptoms* are: a tense enlarged abdomen; considerable thirst; pulse very irregular, and bowels in the same condition.

Post-mortem Appearance.—Liver two or three times its natural size, and consisting of a mass of coagulated blood.

Treatment.—Laxatives combined with diuretics, and food in small quantities.

Degeneration

signifies a change for the worse—*degradation*—in the intimate composition of the solids or fluids of the body. In pathological anatomy it means the change which occurs in the structure of an organ when transformed into fat, for example, or into a matter essentially morbid. Degeneration is very difficult to diagnose, and its existence can only be ascertained by watching carefully the changes it undergoes. You will perceive yellowness of the visible mucous membranes and changeable appetite. The animal seems at times to recover, but is again thrown back, and eventually death takes place.

Treatment consists in proper attention to diet, keeping the bowels in regular working order.

The Pancreas.

This organ secretes the *pancreatic juice*, which resembles the saliva. When this juice is mixed with amylaceous matters, it converts them into dextrin and glucose. Its great function appears, however, to be to emulsify fatty matters by virtue of a peculiar albuminoid principle, *pancreatin*, which it contains, and is coagulable by heat or alcohol. It also dissolves albuminous substances. The pancreatic juice of the pig has been given in the form of emulsion with the fat of beef stirred in milk to consumptive patients, and an emulsion with cod-liver oil is similarly prescribed. The diseases of this organ do not manifest their presence by plain or intelligible signs; it is only after death that we discover them.

The Spleen.

The only disease of any consequence that affects this organ is called splenic apoplexy, the consideration of which we will enter into when we describe the Blood-diseases.

DISEASES OF THE ORGANS OF RESPIRATION.

Respiration is a function proper to all animals, the object of which is to bring the materials of the blood—the mixture of the venous blood with lymph and chyle—into contact with the atmospheric air, in order that they may acquire the vivifying qualities which belong to arterial blood. The organs for executing this function are, in the mammalia, birds, and reptiles, the *lungs*. In man, the respiration consists of mechanical and chemical phenomena. The mechanical are *inspiration* and *expiration*; the chemical phenomena consisting in the formation of a certain quantity of carbonic acid, the absorption of a part of the oxygen of the air, and the disengagement of a quantity of water in the state of vapour. In the healthy condition the respiration is easy, gentle, regular, and without noise, and in cattle should be from about ten to twelve per minute.

The air of respiration has been divided into, *first*, the residual, or that which cannot be expelled from the lungs, but remains after a full and forcible expiration; *secondly*, the supplementary or reserve air, or that which can be expelled by a forcible expiration after an ordinary exhaling; *thirdly*, the breath, tidal or breathing air; and, *fourthly*, the complementary or complemental air, or that which can be inhaled after an ordinary inspiration.

The diseases of the organs of respiration and the air-passages are for the most part inflammatory in their nature, and may affect the parts within the nose separately or collectively. When it affects the nose, it is called catarrh; when the pharynx, it is termed pharyngitis; when the larynx, laryngitis. These diseases may occur separately, but they are, as a rule, found collectively. Thus, in simple catarrh we generally have the larynx and pharynx implicated. The inflammation, however, does not content itself by remaining in these organs, but descends into the bronchial tubes, thus producing bronchitis. When it attacks the lung substance it is termed pneumonia; but when the covering membrane of the lungs is only affected, it is called pleurisy. It is an established fact that inflammation has always a tendency to descend, the reason being that the same membrane lines the whole passage.

By an epizootic disease is meant a disease that prevails in a country or certain portions of a country at the same time, and may appear at any season. It is the same in nature as an epidemic in man, those animals that are of a weak constitution being more liable to attack. In all epizootic diseases the weakest are the first attacked; what benefit, then, can be acquired from depletion? Instead of this, we should use every exertion to assist nature to overcome the diseases.

The inflammatory diseases that affect these organs are of two distinct kinds; namely, one which is characterised by highly irritative fever; the other is of a typhoid or debilitating nature. The former is brought on by accidental causes—such as overdriving, exposure, or in twenty other different ways; the latter by epizootic causes which we cannot account for. At the same time almost all epizootic diseases are accompanied by fever of a typhoid nature. These are facts well worthy of remembrance.

The general causes of inflammatory disease in the respiratory organs are, then, simple and typhoid in their nature. The same causes will, however, produce different diseases in different animals—in some, throat affections; others, bronchitis; others, pleurisy; and others, pneumonia. This is due entirely to the varied constitutions of the animals. These facts bring us to the conclusion that there is among cattle a dissimilarity of constitution, which so modifies these causes that different effects result.

Again, whenever diseases of the air-passages and lungs assume an epizootic form, they become more and more typhoid in their character in proportion to their prevalence.

Again, many of these diseases exhibit similar signs, which require to be very carefully watched and intelligently noticed in order that we may arrive at a correct diagnosis as to the seat of the complaint. Thus, in catarrh, the cough is loud and coarse, and accompanied or followed by sneezing. In bronchitis the cough is shorter, more sudden, and painful, while the frequency and state of the respirations must also be considered. If they are hurried, it indicates some interference in the oxidation of the blood; this is also accompanied by sounds which have to be distinguished by the ear in order properly to understand them.

Catarrh, or Common Cold,

consists in inflammation in the upper parts of the mucous membrane of the nose and throat. It is commonly an affection of but little consequence in its simple form, but is apt to relapse and become chronic. Catarrh is characterised by cough, thirst, lassitude, fever, watery eyes, with increased secretion of mucus from the air-passages. Cold air or any sudden change of temperature induces sneezing and coughing; the animal becomes dull and refuses to feed; difficulty in swallowing ensues; breathing and pulse get hurried; there is congestion of the capillary blood-vessels, which become dilated, the blood now flowing sluggishly through them; the redness increases; mouth hot and muzzle dry; urine scanty and high-coloured; bowels constipated; fæces hard and glazed; irregularity of the temperature of the body; ears and horns cold and hot alternately; legs in the same condition; cough easily excited.

Treatment.—In the simple form, the duration is from three days to a week. Allow plenty of pure fresh air; clothe the body according to the season of the year, and make the patient otherwise as comfortable as you possibly can: put nitre in the water given as drink; steam the head and throat. As a rule, this is all that will be required.

Laryngitis, or Inflammation of the Larynx.

This organ, properly speaking, is the voice apparatus, and is situated at the upper part of the windpipe, with which it communicates. It is moved by a number of muscles, and lined by a mucous membrane having certain membranous reflexions, constituting the superior and inferior ligaments of the glottis. The larynx is destined to give passage to air in the act of respiration, and to impress upon it certain modifications. Its dimensions vary in different animals. The pathological changes that take place in this ailment are congestion, then exudation leading to effusion; this causes a muco-purulent discharge, which proceeds from the nostrils, and is of a deepish yellow or greenish colour, thick and void of odour; the head is kept in a fixed straight line, as movement causes pain. The patient will not partake of food; the cough is harsh and husky; the respiration is not much interfered with, but the pulse may be weak. The duration of the disease is generally about thirteen or fourteen days, when the patient generally recovers. A cough, however, is often left,. after all the other symptoms have disappeared, which is liable to become chronic.

Treatment.—Attend to the diet in the first stages; give sloppy food of a good supporting nature, with nitre and tartar-emetic; steam the head and throat well, and give belladonna and nitre, of each one drachm, night and morning. Should the cough continue, either insert a seton between the lower jaws or apply an active blister.

The Trachea, or Windpipe,

is a cylindrical fibro-cartilaginous and membranous tube, which runs from the larynx to the lungs, where it divides into two branches, called the bronchiæ: these separate, one proceeding to the right lung and the other to the left. The function of this pipe is to convey air to the lungs. It is also liable to inflammation, which may consist in an extension of the disease affecting the throat. The symptoms and treatment are much the same as for laryngitis.

Bronchitis, or Inflammation of the Bronchial Tubes,

is a common and likewise serious disease. Some cases of inflammation of the lungs are accompanied by it, and *vice versâ*. This is often observed in cases of bronchitis terminating in inflammation or pneumonia, although it may exist as an independent disease, which may be contracted either through epizootic or accidental causes. When by the former, it is accompanied by intense prostration; but if arising from the latter, the prostration is not so great.

In bronchitis the mucous membranes of all the tubes are inflamed, though this seems to originate in the two primary ones. As a consequence of this inflammatory process, lymph is formed, and sometimes pus, accompanied by a great amount of mucus. The air passing downwards becomes mixed with it, hence the frothy appearance which it always presents.

You will now perceive that this collection of fluid in the air-tubes must impede the current of air: as a result, the blood cannot be purified as before; this hastens debility. In fact, the strength of the animal depends upon the free passage of pure air into the lungs for the purification of the blood. When blood is propelled by the heart to the lungs, it is for the express purpose of having it purified, and unless it is purified it stops there; hence the origin of congestion of the lungs.

Symptoms of bronchitis are invariably ushered in by a cough, which is short, dry, and husky; this gradually becomes prolonged, hoarse, and painful. The animal tries to close its mouth in order to prevent the coughing. Sympathetic fever present; mouth and muzzle hot and dry; ears, horns, and legs alternately hot and cold; pulse soft and compressible; respiration quickened and shallow, from twenty-three to thirty per minute. If you place your ear to the side of the chest just behind the shoulder-blade, you will hear the air passing into the lungs, giving a sound as of a gentle breeze if the animal is healthy; but in bronchitis the passage of air is obstructed by the accumulation of mucus. The patient never attempts to eat, but will endeavour to drink; this always excites cough. He rarely lies down, and the fæces are hard and glazy. The urine is scanty and high-coloured. Death may occur in three or four days, but as a rule he recovers in about three or four weeks.

Treatment.—Remove the patient into a cool house apart from other animals, then clothe the body and bandage the legs. Administer two ounces of sweet nitre with ten drops of Fleming's tincture of aconite three times a day. Apply hot fomentations to the sides and chest. If the cough is harassing, give belladonna, one drachm, three times a day.

Stimulants are very useful, and ought to be employed say twice daily. Should bronchitis run on to pneumonia or inflammation of the lungs, there is little hope of recovery.

Hoose in Calves.

This disease is dependent upon the presence in the lower parts of the bronchial tube of small thread-like worms, called *Filaria bronchialis*.

Parasites are plants which attach themselves to other plants, and animals which live in or on the bodies of other animals, so as to subsist at their expense. They are common in autumn, sometimes in spring, and abound in old low-lying pastures in the Midland and Southern Counties of England. They are also found in woods where the herbage is coarse and the drainage bad. Calves are subject to this disease up to one year old, but rarely suffer from it when fed on young grasses, it being in the rough grass that the ova find shelter. They are then taken up with the food and transmitted through the circulation to the lungs, where they claim a special habitation; here they are developed. They do not, however, produce inflammation, but they obstruct the egress and ingress of air.

The *Symptoms* are seldom developed suddenly. The animal appears not to be thriving; there is frequent cough, which increases in severity, being always worst when the animal is thirsty or moved about. This causes great distress and difficulty in breathing, accompanied with general dulness. The appetite becomes impaired or entirely lost; the animal loses condition; separates itself from the rest; stands with its back arched; heaving at the flanks. Owing to impaired respiration, the blood cannot be properly purified. The result is total debility, and death in about a week or a fortnight.

Treatment.—Some people administer medicines by the nose, thinking it must have an efficacious effect upon the worms in the lungs. I have seen the experiment tried by a quack professor, who not only succeeded in terminating the parasites' existence, but effectually relieved the poor calf from its troubles in about twenty minutes by choking it. You may employ inhalations of chlorine gas, but half an ounce of turpentine in three or four ounces of castor-oil for a calf six months old, given in the morning when the animal is fasting, and repeated every two or three days until the cough ceases, will generally be all that is required. The turpentine, being volatile, is readily absorbed by the blood, and is then carried into the lungs, where it exercises a fatal influence upon the worms. What becomes of these parasites after they are dead is not well known. They are either coughed up or become absorbed by the blood. Attend to the animal's comfort, giving easily digested food, along with an allowance of good oil-cake.

Structure of the Lungs.

The lungs of quadrupeds have a very complicated structure. In fact, it may be looked upon as not only one lung, but thousands assembled together. One lobule possesses the same structure as the whole lung of a frog. It is simply a sac into which the bronchi open. The anterior portion presents dilatations, and is more vascular than the posterior, which is round. These dilatations are not true cells, but open spaces which increase the area of the lungs, and therefore increase the space for the blood-vessels to ramify, thus facilitating the interchange of gases from the blood-vessels and inspired air. The common cavity into which the bronchi open is called the vestibule or infundibulum, while all the cells in the vestibule communicate freely with one another.

The air-cells have a basement membrane, and are covered by a layer of ciliated epithelium, which is very fine, for the interchange of air. The shape of the air-cells varies, the general form being irregular. The lungs consist entirely of fine elastic tissue, with a small proportion of areolar tissue; between these coverings, then, and the lobules is a rich plexus of blood-vessels. The lungs are supplied with blood directly from the heart in the first instance, for the double purpose of purifying the fluid and nourishing those organs. Physiologists have given the term "circulation" to the motion of the blood through the different vessels of the body,—to that function by which the blood, setting out from the left ventricle of the heart by its impulse, is distributed to every part of the body by the arteries and on through the capillaries, returning to the heart by the veins. All animals intended by the Great Constructor for active exertion possess large lungs in proportion to their body. In the cow these organs are of a whitish colour, and in the calf grey. Investing the lungs we have two diaphanous perspirable membranes called the pleuræ, which line each side of the chest, and are reflected thence upon each lung. Like other serous membranes (to which class they belong), each represents a sac without an aperture. That portion of the pleuræ which lines the *parietes* of the chest is called *pleura costalis*, and that portion which covers the lungs is called *pleura pulmonalis*.

Pneumonia, or Inflammation of the Lungs.

In health the lungs are highly elastic, and when put into water they float, crepitating when pressed between the finger and thumb. In pneumonia the state of the lungs is the reverse of what they are in health; their substance becomes of a reddish-brown colour, ultimately changing to grey, and when put into water will sink.

Pathological Appearances.—First, in the scarlet stage there is a period of increased vascularity; this is called the period of congestion, or sanguineous engorgement. Secondly, when the disease is fully confirmed, the lungs are of a reddish-brown colour, and sink in water; this is called the stage of red hepatisation. The third and last stage is called grey hepatisation, when the lungs are denser and more solid. These three stages are often found existing in one lung at the same time, the lowest part of the lung being usually the worst. Pneumonia does not always attack both lungs at once; the right lung, as a rule, is invariably the one affected first, but in all severe cases they are both implicated. The question may here be asked, How does this occur? But it is one not easily answered. The right lung, of course, is larger, contains more air, and consequently has more blood-vessels than the left one. Why pneumonia should select this lung first for attack, I am unable to explain. It is the same in pleurisy.

The causes that are in operation to produce this disease are similar to those which bring on catarrh, as inflammation has always a tendency to descend. Pneumonia is, therefore, caused by any irritating matter passing down the bronchial tubes into the lung substance. It is ushered in first by a shivering fit, more or less violent according to the nature of the attack; the breathing becomes accelerated and laborious, the mouth hot and dry, and the mucous membranes red and congested. Cough is not an invariable symptom, but when it is present it is full and free, and not so painful as it is in bronchitis. If both lungs are attacked, the inflammation is generally posteriorly; but if only one lung be affected, it may be inflamed throughout its whole extent. The expired air will feel warmer; the breathing becomes heavy and laboured; coldness of all the extremities then sets in, while the body is often bedewed with perspiration. On examination with your ear at the side, you will hear a peculiar crepitating sound; this may be succeeded shortly by a rasping, rumbling noise. The affected portion of the lung now becomes consolidated, when the respiratory murmur ceases, and on percussion or tapping the side with your hand a dull sound is produced.

This disease may terminate in resolution or recovery, and the patient be convalescent in the second week; but in unfavourable cases, where death occurs, this event may take place in about twelve or fourteen days from the commencement of the attack.

The Post-mortem Appearances reveal the fact that the lungs are completely hepatised, or converted into a liver-like substance. They have become engorged with effused matters, so that they are no longer pervious to the air; and are now said to be hepatised, which is the final stage of pneumonia.

Treatment.—The immediate and constant application of hot fomentations is positively essential.

Let these be applied without intermission if you desire the patient's recovery. If the pulse is active and feverish, as in all probability it will be, give fourteen drops of Fleming's tincture of aconite, repeated at intervals of two hours, until the mouth becomes moist and cool. No advantage will be derived from exposing the animal to intense cold pure air. Clothe the body and bandage the limbs, which ought to be well hand-rubbed before you apply the bandages, in order to assist the restoration of the circulation to these parts. Should the patient's thirst be great, mix nitre with the water given to drink. This prevents the blood from coagulating and dissolves the fibrin. As a most important part of the treatment, give stimulants and food of an easily digestible nature. When the inflammatory process has subsided, give mineral and vegetable tonics.

Abscesses in the Lungs

may occur as a result of bronchitis or pneumonia. That part of the lung surrounding the abscess is clean and healthy; the bronchial tubes may communicate with it, when its contents are thrown up. The animal does not thrive; there is a cough present, while the skin is usually hide-bound, with a disagreeable fetid breath. The patient has no appetite, and ultimately dies. *Treatment*, none available.

Pleurisy, or Inflammation of the Pleuræ.

As already stated, the pleura covers the lungs and lines the inside of the chest. It is a serous membrane, secreting serum, not mucus; is much thinner than a mucous membrane, and, like it, consists of several parts.

First, we have a layer of epithelial scales.

Secondly, there is a limitary membrane, which is very thin.

Thirdly, the sub-pleural or fibrous tissue contains no follicles or villi, like the mucous membrane.

A serous membrane has a more mechanical function to fulfil than a mucous membrane; it secretes a fluid to prevent friction.

Now, in a state of health the lungs are continually rubbing against the ribs; this friction, however, is not felt, as the parts are all kept moist. The pleura of an old animal is as smooth and bright as that of a young one.

Pleurisy is a common disease in all animals that we have to do with. We may have it independently of any other complaint, yet it is often combined with pneumonia, and *vice versâ*.

It is a disease in which the inflammatory process is very distinctly marked. I think no disease is better defined than this one, for in all cases there is a structural change corresponding to the intensity of the inflammation. When exudation takes place, lymph collects on the surface. This exudation is most copious on the pleura covering the ribs and the diaphragm,—sometimes half an inch thick, getting gradually less as we proceed to the back.

Pleurisy mostly begins in the costal region, at its lower surface, extending upwards. This disease attacks both sides, but has a preference, like pneumonia, for the right one, which is generally the worst. It frequently causes death in cattle when only one side is affected.

The Morbid Changes of Pleurisy.

First, we have the membrane reddened; a small patch on the lower surface of the pleura appears; this expands upwards. Succeeding this we have exudation, causing a thickening of the membrane on its surface, the consequence of which is that the pleura looks thick, muddy, and rough. If this exudation is rubbed off, the redness in the sub-pleural or fibrous texture is plainly seen through the limitary membrane.

This collection of lymph necessarily causes the pleuræ to be rough, and when they rub one against the other, a sharp, darting pain is produced. This stage may be reached in from six to eight hours.

When the disease is prolonged, the exudation becomes more and more abundant, the result being that we have a quantity of water collecting in the chest; and as this liquid always seeks its own level, it sinks to the floor of the chest, filling up the vacant cavity.

The lungs now float upon this fluid, and as it accumulates it prevents them from expanding. An idea may be formed as to this feature of the disease when I state that twelve gallons of water have been taken from the chest of one animal.

It not unfrequently happens that when an animal is tapped no water makes its appearance. This is most likely due to the lymph being in great abundance. I have known cases of pneumonia mistaken for pleurisy, the patient being tapped for water when none was present.

Symptoms.—First, it may be remarked that pleurisy is far more painful than pneumonia, therefore we have more fever. The reason of this increased pain is, that in pleurisy the inflamed parts cannot expand like the lungs, but are put on their utmost stretch. This disease is often announced by a shivering fit, caused by a determination of blood inwardly. When this fit passes off, inflammatory fever commences, and the patient begins to blow. Sometimes griping pains are manifested. At the beginning of an attack we cannot tell whether it is to be a case of pneumonia or pleurisy. In a few hours, however, the distinct symptoms show themselves, when there can no longer be any mistake.

There may or may not be a cough at first; the

breathing is quick and laboured in a peculiar way, and the inspiration rather prolonged, or doubled. This is distinctly seen in genuine cases. If it is not prolonged, it will be interrupted and catching : this is due to the patient stretching his lungs as slowly as possible, in order prevent pain.

Then another prominent symptom appears, which is shown by a muscular ridge extending along the ends of the ribs to the flank, while the belly is tucked up. The cause of this ridge is owing to the animal, in breathing, keeping his ribs stationary. He is afraid to move them, so the abdominal muscles are brought into action in order to prevent the pain. The pulse is quick, small, hard, and wiry, seeming to throw your finger off the artery. There is great irritative fever, accompanied by obstruction of the lungs. These are obvious signs in all cases of pleurisy. In addition to these we shall enumerate others. If you place your ear to the right side, you hear in the very early stage a creaking sound. In the second stage a rubbing sound is heard, showing that the two roughened surfaces of the pleuræ are rubbing one against the other. If you apply pressure between the ribs with your finger, it causes great· pain. The animal turns unwillingly, and in doing so utters an agonised grunt. The patient frequently looks to his side, endeavouring to direct your attention to the seat of the disease by touching it with his nose : this is a silent but forcible appeal for help, and not easily withstood. He will also stand with his nose outstretched, having a sinking eye and drooping head.

If there is a mitigation of the symptoms about the third or fourth day in pneumonia, it is a good sign; but in pleurisy we frequently find the patient suddenly looking very lively just about this period. The fever and breathing are not so intense; the coat looks better, smooth and glossy; therefore we are apt to be misled. There is one sign, however, that never deceives us, and that is the pulse: if the pulse be quicker and softer, the animal is not better, but worse. By this time the inflammation has extended over a great amount of surface, and the quickened and soft pulse proves that the vessels are relieved by exudation, which speedily tells upon the system at large. This is the time to make use of your ears by applying them to the patient's sides and noting the different sounds. By-and-by the breathing gets quicker and shallower, the air seeming to go less into the chest; heaving at the flanks becomes more pronounced. The eye now looks pearly bright and the skin glossy, with a peculiar wasting away of the muscles over the surface of the ribs.

No one can be deceived by such symptoms as these, even if he pay no attention to the pulse. Every day the exudation increases as the disease progresses, until at last we scarcely hear any respiratory murmur at all. The breathing now becomes more and more rapid, and superficial dropsy under the abdomen takes place.

On percussion, dulness is observed as high as the water has reached; in this stage both sides are sure to be affected, but the water will not be on a level in either side, as in the horse, unless the whole pleura is implicated. There is also a gurgling sound, but it is not to be relied upon, for we have it occurring in pneumonia. Some authors class this as a first-rate symptom, but it is well known that a sound can never be generated without air being in the chest. This may be shown by placing a bell in a jar, when you will be surprised that no sound is heard if you first exhaust the air in it by an air-pump.

Favourable signs are, the pulse losing its wiry tone and getting slower towards the fourth or fifth day; we may then entertain hopes of recovery, for the breathing is getting deeper and the fever less. Often after an attack of pleurisy we find adhesions taking place between the lungs and pleura of the chest; but this does not cause much harm unless the adhesions are large. At other times, collections of white spots are formed on the costal pleura.

This disease, then, on the whole, is more fatal than pneumonia, unless proper remedies are applied in the very early stage; if it gets beyond that, it is very difficult to manage.

Treatment in every way similar to pneumonia. Some approve of the tapping remedy, others do not.

I have never seen any good results follow from its adoption.

When pleurisy destroys life, it effects this by copious exudation. If this exudation is only about one-third the depth of the chest, the water can be absorbed by giving tonics and diuretics; but when the liquid extends half-way, little more can be done except tapping, which is very unlikely to succeed.

Pleuro-Pneumonia.

This disease is very common. It occurs in all kinds of cattle, and at all ages. It is a peculiarly inflammatory disease of a low typhoid character, and affects the upper lobules of the lungs first. All authorities are now agreed as to the contagious nature it possesses. The definition of *contagion* may be summed up as the transmission of a disease from one affected person or animal to another by direct or indirect contact. This term has also been applied by some to the action of miasmata arising from dead animal or vegetable matter, &c., but in this sense it is now abandoned. Contagious diseases are produced either by a virus capable of originating them by inoculation, as in small-pox, cow-pox, hydrophobia, &c.; or by miasmata proceeding from a sick individual, as in plague, typhus fever, measles, or scarlatina. However, medical men are by no means unanimous in deciding which diseases are contagious and which are not. It seems probable that a disease may be contagious under certain conditions and circumstances, and not under others. A case of common fever arising from ordinary causes, such as cold, if the patient be kept in a close, foul, ill-ventilated situation, may be converted into a disease capable of producing emanations which may excite a similar disease in those exposed to them. Contagion and infection are generally esteemed the same. Frequently, however, the former is applied to diseases not produced by contact, as measles, scarlet fever, &c.; while *infection* is used for those that require positive contact to reproduce them, such as itch, skin diseases, &c.; and conversely, diseases which cannot be produced in any other way than by contagion are said to have their origin in *specific contagion;* and those which are produced by contagion, and yet are supposed to be sometimes owing to other causes, are said to arise from common contagion.

A few years ago it was believed that pleuro-pneumonia never appeared in home-bred cattle. Some say it is due to atmospheric influences; others again declare that it is caused by bad ventilation, exposure to draughts, &c., the affected animals having a predisposition to take it. Others think it an epizootic brought on by contagion, favoured by exciting or predisposing causes; with which theory I entirely agree.

Pleuro-pneumonia has attacked cattle from time

immemorial. It is believed to be the same disease that prevailed in the year 1693. It was imported into this country from Holland in the year 1842, spreading rapidly throughout the whole kingdom. Some declared that it assumed two forms, simple or non-contagious and contagious. It is a low typhoid disease, in which lymph is thrown out in considerable quantity, the exudation assuming the form of pus corpuscles, when interlobular pneumonia begins simultaneously. The inflammation extends to the parenchyma, and runs three or four stages. In the first place, there is passive congestion, in which the veins become congested. This is followed by an inflammatory exudation and formation of lymph. Succeeding this we have hepatisation, or that condition of the lungs in which they are gorged with effused matters. As the disease progresses, a fluid is exuded and taken up by the capillaries; the blood in these vessels becomes decomposed, and black spots begin to be observed in the surrounding tissues. As the disease advances the lungs become heavy and gangrenous. If you cut the diseased lung through in the third stage, the whole of the organ will be found diseased. If in the second stage, one-half will be found in the same condition; and if in the first stage, the upper border only is implicated; this shows plainly enough that the disease commences in this portion of the lung. The pleura pulmonalis, being also involved, rubs against the opposing pleura during respiration, producing that peculiar sound which is heard by placing your ear to the animal's side. In milk-cows the udder and teats are painful to the touch, and the milk, if any, of a frothy nature; there is a short, shallow, painful cough; breathing quickened; pulse quick, small, and weak; the nose is poked out; the nostrils distended and drawn up; the muzzle dry; appetite suspended; secretion of milk fails; lastly, the characteristic unmistakable grunt is given forth, which when once you hear you will never forget. The back is arched.; the coat rough and staring; eyes prominent and bright, but towards the termination of the disease they are shallow and sunk; wasting of the muscles along the sides; hide-bound; horns, ears, and legs cold; heaving or lifting at the flanks; and generally diarrhœa in the later stages, the fæces having a very fetid smell, death occurring from want of oxygen.

Terminations are recovery, or sloughing and death. When an animal seems to recover, and afterwards dies of another disease, the lungs are found hardened and solidified; therefore it cannot be regarded as true recovery.

Treatment.—According to the Act, we are not at liberty to treat this disease, and there can be no doubt that the stamping-out process is the best remedy for such a contagious affection.

Tuberculosis.

Tubercle is a tumour arising in the substance of any organ. In pathological anatomy, the term is generally given to a species of degeneration which consists of an opaque matter of a pale yellow colour, having in its crude condition a consistence analogous to that of concrete albumen. It subsequently becomes soft and friable, and gradually acquires a consistence and appearance similar to those of pus. Tubercles may be developed in different parts of the body;—for example, in the tissue of the alimentary canal; in serous structures, as the pleuræ, peritoneum, and arachnoid; in the liver, kidneys, spleen, and lungs; but they are most frequently observed in the lungs and mesentery.

Some authors class tubercles among the accidental tissues, which have no resemblance to the natural tissues, and which never exist except in consequence of morbid action. But the prevalent doctrine at the present day is that they are the products of a scrofulous degeneration. Tubercle is, in other words, merely a local expression of a constitutional scrofulous affection. The view has also been held by some writers that tubercle is a degeneration of previously existing structures, whether physiological or pathological; by others, that it is a morbid exudation, a new formation. Again, according to some authorities, although tubercle is a result of the death

F

of healthy or diseased tissues, the local process—tuberculosis—also results in the exudation of a material during a *tuberculous inflammation*, such material undergoing a kind of organisation, succeeded by death, and by its breaking and shrivelling up into a tubercle; this gradual change being termed "tuberculisation." But tubercle is produced independently of inflammation, although the latter may be excited around a tubercle or a mass of tubercles, and thus promote their further development, or their progress towards softening and destruction of structure. When tubercles in any organ are few in number, they may pass to the state of permanent induration without danger to the patient; but when they are very numerous, they usually cause serious mischief.

Symptoms.—In the early stage we have a simple cough; dulness; quick, weak pulse; gradual emaciation; hide-bound skin, which becomes dry and often infested with parasites; the cough becomes more painful; diarrhœa sets in, with watery effusion from the mouth. Cows affected with it yield a large quantity of bluish milk, stand with their back arched, and have a ewe-necked appearance; appetite capricious, while cough becomes continuous.

Treatment.—Very uncertain. Give food rich in starchy and fatty matters; generous diet; comfortable housing; plenty of fresh air; mineral tonics, lime-water, oil-cakes, &c.

DISEASES AFFECTING THE CIRCULATORY ORGANS.

The diseases affecting the heart are distinct and idiopathic, although they accómpany, as a rule, rheumatism, distemper, pneumonia, pleuro-pneumonia, &c. They are, however, of more frequent occurrence in old than in young animals.

Pericarditis, or Inflammation of the Covering of the Heart.

This is probably the proper appellation for most of those cases which have received the names of carditis, cardo-pericarditis, &c.

This disease is seen in all our domestic animals, and is of more common occurrence in cattle than in the horse. The causes which give rise to it are generally those which produce disease in the respiratory organs, such as cold, alteration of the temperature, &c.

The *Symptoms* are, pulse accelerated and irritable; great fever and anxiety; panting; dulness; eyes bright and prominent; great unwillingness to move; the patient exhibits great suffering when you press your finger between the ribs; distinct vibrating pulsations; limbs, horns, and ears cold. As the disease advances, you can scarcely hear the heart beat; on listening, however, you hear a distinct friction-sound, consequently it is often very difficult to decide between this disease and pleurisy. *Post-mortem* examinations reveal the heart firm and contracted; veins full of dark blood; lungs congested; spots of ecchymosis on the heart's surface, with thickening of the covering membrane and the formation of false ones.

Treatment.—Give belladonna and digitalis, as these agents tranquillise the heart and diminish the calibre of the blood-vessels, more especially if they are administered along with salines. Half-drachm doses of either medicine twice a day will be sufficient. Apply mustard embrocations to the chest, hand-rub the legs, and attend to the diet and general comfort. As a sequel we often find

Hydrops Pericarde, or Dropsy of the Heart's Bag.

Symptoms.—Small weak pulse, often irregular; heart's beat feebly felt over a large surface; frequently diarrhœa and dropsical swellings.

Treatment. — Give diuretics, tonics, and stimulants to support the system, and keep the animal perfectly quiet.

Dilatation of the Heart

is found to be an accompaniment of pericarditis, and consists in the softening of the walls of the heart, the symptoms of which are similar to those characteristic of pericarditis.

Cause.—The heart being called into inordinate action or motion.

Treatment.—If accompanied by disease of the lungs, give stimulants, diuretics, good food, and fresh air.

Hypertrophy of the Heart.

Owing to nutrition being performed with great activity, the heart at length acquires unusual bulk. Hypertrophy is also sometimes used to denote a simple dilatation.

Symptoms.—The impulse of the heart is greatly increased; pulse full, strong, and irregular.

Treatment.—Keep the animal free from excitement and attend to the diet.

Atrophy of the Heart.

This is a rare malady, in which the muscles become so greatly atrophied that they cannot perform their function. It may take place in one or more of the cavities. It occurs mostly in old animals, and is not very well understood till death occurs. The impulse will be much weaker than when the animal is in health.

No treatment available.

Fatty Degeneration of the Heart.

This disease is also commonly met with in old animals, and is an unusual deposition of fat on the heart; by some presumed occasionally to be a true adipose degeneration of the substance of the heart.

Symptoms.—Intermittent pulse, great difficulty in moving, palpitation, &c.

Treatment of little use.

Rupture of the Heart

may occur in a healthy as well as in a diseased animal, but it is generally met with in those that suffer from fatty degeneration. It is often the result of over-exertion.

No remedy.

Diseases of the Arteries.

Aneurism signifies a tumour produced by the dilatation of an artery; but it has been extended to lesions of arteries as well as to dilatations of the heart. There are various kinds. The following are the principal disease :—

First, When the blood which forms the tumour is enclosed within the dilated coats of the artery. This is true aneurism.

Second, When the blood has escaped from the opened artery, it is called spurious or false aneurism, the latter being divided into three varieties—1st,

Diffused false aneurism, which occurs immediately after the division or rupture of an artery, and consists of an extravasation of blood into the areolar texture of the part; 2d, Circumscribed false aneurism, in which the blood issues from the vessel some time after the receipt of the wound, and forms for itself a sac in the neighbouring areolar tissue; 3d, Aneurism by anastomosis, which may arise from the simultaneous wounding of an artery and a vein, the arterial blood passing into the vein and producing a varicose state of it, or by an increase of arterial tissue and a dilatation and elongation of arteries. The term *cirsoid* is employed when the trunks of the larger vessels are involved, and *aneurism by anastomosis* when the smaller vessels and capillaries are affected.

Aneurisms have also been divided into internal and external. The internal are situated in the great cavities, and occur in the heart and great vessels of the chest, abdomen, &c. Their diagnosis is difficult, and they are inaccessible to treatment. The external aneurisms are situated at the exterior of the head, neck, and limbs, and are distinctly pulsatory.

Treatment.—Tie the artery where practicable.

Diseases of the Veins.

Phlebitis, or inflammation of the veins, is the most common. It sometimes follows the operation of blood-letting, and extends from the small wound made in that operation to the neighbouring parts of the venous system. The symptoms are, first, inflammation in the punctured part, after which there occurs a knotty, tense, painful chord, following the direction of the vessel, and accompanied by more or less fever, according to the extent of the inflammation. It may terminate by resolution, suppuration, ulceration, or gangrene. Sometimes, when a clot forms in a vein, and the vessel becomes permanently obliterated, the clot and vein ultimately contract so as to form a firm cord; in this case it constitutes adhesive phlebitis.

Treatment.—Foment, poultice; keep the patient quiet, and heal up; give a dose of physic, and attend to the general comfort.

DISEASES OF THE URINARY ORGANS.

These organs comprise the kidneys, bladder, uterus, and urethra.

The kidneys secrete from the blood the fluid called urine. These organs are situated in the loins, the one on the right being placed a little further forward than that on the left. The kidneys of the ox are less than those of any other animal in proportion to their size. The healthy urine of the ox is alkaline in its action, and when allowed to cool it forms a sediment. The composition of the urine of the ox is about 928 parts of water in 1000 parts of urine, the remainder being composed of matters held in solution. This urine is an excrementitial fluid, secreted, as shown above, by the kidneys, and transmitted by them to the ureters, which convey it slowly but in a continuous manner into the bladder, where it remains deposited until the uneasiness caused by its accumulation excites a desire to void it. The excretion of the fluid takes place through the urethra, and is caused by the united action of the abdominal muscles and diaphragm and the contraction of the fibrous coat of the bladder.

In all internal diseases appertaining to the ox and cow, the kidneys are frequently brought into requisition in order to discharge from the system the deleterious residue caused by the various complaints.

Diabetes

is a disease characterised by great augmentation, and often manifest alteration, in the secretion of urine, with excessive thirst and progressive emaciation. It may be looked upon simply as a superabundant discharge of limpid urine. Where the disease is situated is not very clearly defined, but the whole system of nutrition seems to be morbidly implicated. Now this extraordinary discharge must be made at the expense of the system; but on dissection no morbid appearance is met with sufficient to enable us to fix the seat of this distressing affection. In the human subject all the remedies tried have signally failed.

Symptoms.—Indigestion; pulse weak; great quantities of urine voided, which is usually clear; no appetite; hidebound skin; great thirst; dry coat, with great irritation of the urinary and genital organs, accompanied by constipation.

Treatment.—Change the food entirely, substituting that which is easily digested; give lime-water along with the drinking-water; also sulphate of iron combined with gentian, and ginger night and morning. If the bowels are costive, give a slight purge in order to move them gently, and keep the patient comfortable.

Nephritis, or Inflammation of the Kidneys.

This is a disease of pretty frequent occurrence in the cow. The most common causes that produce it are the abuse of diuretics, blows over the loins, or the presence of a calculus or stone in the kidneys.

Symptoms.—General sympathetic fever; pulse full and bounding; colicky pains; the animal looks frequently round to her flanks; straddling gait; scanty discharge of urine, which is voided with great pain, and sometimes tinged with blood; belly tucked up; pain across the loins; pulse weak, and breathing hurried.

Treatment.—Administer a good purge of linseed

CYSTITIS, OR INFLAMMATION OF THE BLADDER. 91

oil, as it is the best, with aromatics and sedatives. Apply hot fomentations to the region of the loins. If this is impossible, put on a fresh sheepskin. Clothe the body and legs. Allow plenty of carbonate of soda in the drinking-water, with good sloppy food.

Hæmaturia, or Bloody Urine,

or hæmorrhage from the mucous membrane of the urinary passages. Like other hæmorrhages, it may be active or passive, and may proceed from the kidneys or the urethra. The essential symptoms are blood evacuated by the urethra, preceded by pain in the region of the bladder or kidneys. The treatment to be adopted must consist of cooling lotions, a mild laxative, and carbonate of soda in the drinking-water. If in much pain, give the patient opium. Absolute repose is strictly enjoined.

Cystitis, or Inflammation of the Bladder.

This disease is characterised by a painful discharge of urine. It may affect one or all of the membranes of the bladder, but commonly it is confined to the mucous coat. In the chronic condition cystitis appears in the form of cystirrhœa.

Symptoms.— Great pain; urine evacuated frequently, often accompanied by diarrhœa; straddling gait; and tenderness over the part.

Treatment.—Sedatives. Put a fresh sheepskin over

the loins. Give plenty of pure water; in short, follow nearly the same course as is recommended for the other disorders of the urinary organs.

Rupture of the Bladder

may be caused by a fall, when of course little or nothing can be done. The bladder is liable to cancer and to calculi, the best treatment for which is to consign the animal to the butcher.

DISEASES OF THE GENERATIVE ORGANS.

Ovarian Dropsy.

This is a somewhat rare disease in the domestic animals. It is sometimes seen, however, in the cow, but seldom in calves. It consists of a watery effusion into the womb.

Symptoms.—Distension of the abdomen, which may be distinguished by its position from dropsy in the abdomen. It is sometimes mistaken for pregnancy, but may be diagnosed by the absence of the fœtus, which can be felt on the right side.

Treatment.—Diuretics and good food.

Leucorrhœa, or the Whites.

This is a disease which affects cows a little after conception, or after parturition. It is a more or less abundant discharge of a white, yellowish, or greenish mucus, resulting from acute or chronic inflammation, or from irritation of the membranes lining the genital organs. Leucorrhœa is often attended by pain and disordered digestive functions, causing at times the health of the animal to suffer greatly.

Treatment.—Give a saline purge; inject mild astringent lotions, followed up with tonics.

Inflammation of the Uterus or Womb

is mostly seen after calving, where there has been considerable difficulty in getting away the calf. It frequently occurs in young animals after giving birth to their first calf, and is often accompanied by peritonitis.

Symptoms.—Pulse quick and wiry; breathing hurried; the animal staggers; a blackened fluid is discharged, while the patient utters oft-repeated moans. It is very fatal in cows.

Treatment.—Inject tepid water into the womb at intervals. Apply hot cloths wrung out of boiling water. Give digitalis, opium, nitre, and, as recovery advances, good food and tonics.

Inversion of the Uterus or Womb.

In this case the womb is turned inside out, which can only happen through want of proper caution. It is a fatal accident unless speedily rectified. This must be done by gradually returning the superior part, and elevating the hind legs well. By applying your closed fists get it into its proper situation as quickly as possible. Keep the patient quiet, and give food sparingly.

Parturition.

Labour is the necessary consequence of conception, pregnancy, and the completion of gestation, the cause producing this being the contraction of the uterus and abdominal muscles when the natural term has expired.

The first sign of gestation in the cow is the distension of the abdomen. After the animal has gone some time the calf may be felt by pressing your closed fist into the right side a little above the flank; also by allowing the animal to drink cold water, when you will notice the calf leap; also by examination per rectum, when you can feel it with your hand. The secretion of milk becomes arrested about two months or six weeks before calving; the udder then gradually enlarges, and is filled with colostrum, or the first milk that the udder contains. This fluid possesses more serum and butter and less casein than common milk, and has therefore a laxative effect when the cow is allowed to drink it after calving. The teats get hot, and a relaxation of the ligaments or slipping indicates that delivery is drawing near; the animal evinces great restlessness, moving about, lying down, and rising up. As the labour pains advance the neck of the uterus becomes dilated, and the external membrane of the fœtus is exposed. The animal now stands with the hind limbs apart, the back being arched. The period of gestation in the cow is nine months. In a natural presentation the fore-feet appear first, with the head resting on the knees. On no account be in a hurry to assist a cow when everything is going on well. I well remember an Irishman being interrogated in the following manner:—*Question.*—" What would you do, providing that everything was going on well, and the calf in its natural position?" *Answer.*— " Shure I would go into the house and help the man to drink his whisky." There may be no occasion to follow this bibulous gentleman's advice, but you will certainly err on the safe side by allowing the patient her own time.

There are, however, many and various presentations met with. For example, in twin labour we generally have the first calf in a right position, with the hind-legs of the other presented also; or you may have the hind-legs of one and the head of the other. Always make yourself certain that you seize the fore-legs and the head of the same calf; if not, you must adjust them properly. Again, you may have the fore-legs presented and the head turned back on the shoulder, or it may be down between the fore-legs. You may also have the head presented without the legs, or it may be a back presentation, or a side one, or a breech one; in fact, it is astonishing how various are the attitudes in which they are occasionally placed. Sometimes, owing to enlargement, the head cannot be got through the aperture; in such a case you require to dissect back the skin and remove it in portions; and in some cases this method has to be adopted with the whole calf. When you are compelled to resort to this plan, always secure a cord round the liberated skin, so that you can have a pull at it when required. Never neglect to secure by a cord whatever skin is presented. No doubt many of my readers will say this is all very well on paper, but the successful treatment of a difficult case is not so easily accomplished. The writer has encountered almost every conceivable kind of presentation, and has always undertaken with alacrity to do the utmost for the patient. When you have your animal safely delivered, administer a dose of opening medicine. This is a safe practice, and will prevent any pecuniary loss.

Abortion.

This is the expulsion of the fœtus before the seventh month of utero-gestation, or before it is visible. The causes originate either in the mother or in the calf: those in the mother may be extreme debility, plethora, faulty conformation, violent exercise, fright, &c.; the result in the calf is death, or rupture of the membranes. A cow that has aborted once is liable to do it again, therefore it is better not to run the risk a second time.

DISEASES AFTER CALVING.

The diseases that generally affect the cow after calving were wont to be classified under one distinct head; and even yet many thrust their hasty and ill-timed opinion or verdict upon you with the greatest composure and confidence. Whenever a cow is prostrated after the birth of her calf, the cry is

Parturient Fever.

Now I don't dispute the existence of this malady, but it is well that matters of importance should receive their proper appellations.

The diseases, then, that attack the cow after calving, are, first, parturient fever; secondly, parturient apoplexy; thirdly, parturient paralysis; and fourthly, simple milk fever.

Parturient Fever.—This consists in inflammation of the peritoneum throughout its whole extent, womb and bowels included, accompanied by typhoid fever. It occurs in cows of all ages and under any circumstances, and generally makes its attack from two to four days after calving. When a week has elapsed, an animal may be said to be safe from this malady. It is, however, of most frequent occurrence in young animals, and usually follows labour in a very short space of time. It is often traceable to exposure,

G

and often attacks newly purchased animals that have been driven and knocked about from one place to another without consideration or mercy. How often do we see those poor, exhausted, thirsty, overdriven animals, with the premonitory pains of labour upon them, sink down whenever they enter a friendly abode! In such cases no wonder the fatality is frequent. The animal's vigour, instead of being husbanded, is exhausted, at the very time when it is of the utmost importance that she should have greater strength.

Symptoms of this disease are generally ushered in two or three days after calving, and sometimes sooner. The cow gets restless and uneasy; she has no inclination to eat or to chew the cud. If the milk is scarce, there is great tenderness of the belly and udder. She repeatedly looks round to her flanks, lies down, moans in a painfully expressive manner, stretches out her head, attempts to rise, kicks at her belly with the hind-feet; great fever; eyes staring; ears, horns, and legs cold; pulse at first strong and distinct, it then rises in number of beats, but diminishes in strength; the breathing is quick and laboured. Finally, she lies with head erect, but retains her senses and power of motion until the last.

Cows may labour under this disease for two or three days; but, as a rule, it terminates fatally in forty-eight hours.

Post-mortem Appearances.— Inflammation of the

uterus or womb; both without and within the walls are thickened with mucus, and blackened from extravasated blood; the peritoneal surface is wholly inflamed, and the bowels partake more or less of the same nature, and are studded with lymph, which glues their surfaces together.

Treatment.—If attended to in the early stage, before the symptoms become very acute, there is hope of recovery. A smart active purge must be administered, one that will go straight to its work, such as one pound of linseed-oil or castor-oil; three or four ounces of tincture of opium; twenty croton beans; or instead of this latter agent, one drachm of calomel. If after several hours the medicine fail to operate, renew the oil and opium; give also tepid injections with linseed-oil in them; hot fomentations to the spine; milk often, and turn her repeatedly if she is unable to do so herself; give also powerful stimulants and linseed-tea; and during convalescence attend to her general comfort.

Parturient Apoplexy.—Formerly this name was always, and in fact still is by many, used in a restricted sense to signify the train of phenomena which characterise cerebral apoplexy.

Apoplexy and cerebral hæmorrhage were formerly described as synonymous conditions, under the names of cerebral hæmorrhage, sanguineous apoplexy, &c., characterised by diminution or loss of sensation and mental manifestation, by the cessation, more or less complete, of motion, and by a comatose state, circulation and respiration still continuing. It generally consisted in pressure upon the brain, either from turgescence of vessels or from extravasation of blood. Cerebral apoplexy may occur, however, without any intracranial extravasation of blood, although there is usually partial disease of the cerebral blood-vessels; and cerebral hæmorrhage may not be attended with apoplectiform phenomena.

Parturient Apoplexy

denotes a comatose condition, resulting from pressure on the brain from any cause within the cranium which tends to produce cerebral congestion, such as the immoderate use of stimulants, degeneration of the nervous and vascular structures, and valvular disease of the heart, &c.

The term *congestive apoplexy* has been applied to those cases in which hyperæmia of the brain or its membranes is found after death; or, in other words, a preternatural accumulation of blood in the capillary vessels.

Now the longer this disease is in making its appearance, there is the more chance of the patient's recovery. It generally occurs from two to four days after calving; it never follows abortion, while after the fourth or fifth calf the cow may be said to enjoy immunity from it. It is almost peculiar to wellbred animals and good milkers. It is specially due to the larger quantity of blood which was used for the nutriment of the fœtus before birth, and which was not directed to the proper place or equally distributed, but has found its way to the brain. The bowels are torpid, the udder does not exercise its proper functions, and the blood that it ought to use is arrested in its course to that part. The urine is suppressed; sluggish, almost imperceptible pulse; suppressed breathing; eyes dull; patient staggers and lies down; head turned towards the side, with a comatose condition present.

Treatment.—Administer a brisk active purge followed up with stimulants. When the medicine has operated, the congested parts are immediately relieved. If the patient has reached the comatose state before any remedy has been given, the case is generally hopeless. Apply cold applications to the head, hot cloths to the back; turn the patient frequently; apply friction to the extremities, putting them into a glowing heat, which indicates the return of circulation to those parts. This friction must be kept up. Draw off all milk as it accumulates, relieve the bladder by withdrawing the urine, and make comfortable.

Prevention.—Keep the cow sparingly, before calving, on easily digested soft food; if fat, give a good purge, and keep the bowels in a relaxed condition.

Parturient Paralysis.—Paralysis signifies abolition or great diminution of the voluntary motions, and sometimes cessation in one or more parts of the body. It is said to be local when it affects only a few muscles. When it extends to half the body it is termed paraplegia.

The immediate cause is either by blood effused, or by serum, nervous debility, or by severe straining, &c., at and before calving. The animal loses all control over the hinder extremities. This loss of nervous power is experienced in the bowels as well, hence the great difficulty in getting this function restored. In this disease it signifies little what quantity of medicines you administer so long as the nervous force is suspended, because with this function in absolute repose the organs are lying stationary; therefore, in order to arouse them into action, a powerful stimulant must be given, and repeated at short intervals until the medicine you have administered in the shape of a purge has acted. Combined with whisky, I have attained to great success by the adoption of strychnine in four-grain doses; but this cannot be long continued, as it is a subtle poison, and must be used with great caution. It may, however, be given with safety twice a day in the above quantities. Apply heat and friction to the back; and when once the patient regains her feet, you have little more to fear.

Simple Milk-fever is the last of the series of diseases that imediately attack the cow after calving. It is partly a febrile and partly an inflammatory state of the system, the symptoms of which are tenderness of the udder, breathing accelerated, pulse small and quick, appetite lost.

Treatment.—Give a saline purge; apply friction, such as hand-rubbing, to the abdomen and udder, with nitre in the water given to drink; draw the teats occasionally, and keep her free from cold draughts.

Mammitis, or Inflammation of the Udder,

occurs as a sequel to parturition, and is vulgarly termed a weed. It is due either to cold or imperfect milking, and may be divided into two kinds—superficial and deep-seated. Superficial mammitis is that form where the skin and mucous membrane only are affected. It is said to be deep-seated when the vascular texture is inflamed. In the first form, the skin is thickened, red, hot, and painful, while it feels as if it were bound tightly to the parts beneath. The gland increases in size, and is very sore to the touch, while the milk diminishes and has a curdled appearance. In the second or deep-seated form we may have two or three quarters affected, and at times even the whole udder, while there are hard nodulated swellings in the loose textures. This form is more difficult to treat. It may be produced by blows, such as kicking, by some inhuman, barbarous, cruel wretch; or it may be by the reprehensible practice of allowing the poor creature to carry an overloaded udder in order to present a grand show when offered for sale at markets; or it may be produced by overdriving, or badly treated murrain or foot-and-mouth disease.

Symptoms.—Udder red and swollen, hot and painful; secretion of milk arrested, or nearly so; and when the animal is made to move, she has a peculiar straddling gait.

Treatment.—Apply hot fomentations, and have a strong bandage made, one that will go right round the loins. Make holes in it, in order to pass the teats through; it should be of sufficient breadth to support the heavy swollen udder. Next get some cotton wool or nice soft tow, which you will require to place between the teats and around the udder. With this soft comfortable bandage applied, the owner will be astonished at the rapid relief manifested by the grateful patient. Give also a dose of laxative medicine, and apply plenty of lard, gently yet firmly rubbed into the udder. If the teats are blocked up with curdled milk or any other obstruction, a siphon will have to be passed, which ought to be well oiled before insertion. Should abscesses exist, they will require to be opened; and when gangrene sets in, as it sometimes does, you must resort to amputation, and dress the wound with the ordinary wound-dressing mixtures, such as carbolic oil, &c.

DISEASES OF THE NERVOUS SYSTEM.

Tetanus, or Locked-Jaw,

is so called because it clenches together the jaws. It is a disease of the nervous system, inducing a continued spasmodic contraction of all the voluntary and most of the involuntary muscles of the body. There are few cases in which the muscles about the head and neck are only affected; when such is the case, it is called Trismus. Tetanus is a disease of more frequent occurrence in the bull than in the cow.

Symptoms.—These are singularly alike, whether we notice the disease in man, horse, or bull. It occurs under two distinct forms, traumatic and idiopathic.

By traumatic is meant that kind of tetanus which arises from causes which we can ascertain—such as pricks, outward injuries, &c.

Idiopathic tetanus is that kind which arises without any assignable cause. This distinction, I am afraid, cannot be maintained, for the cogent reasons herewith adduced. As it is now known that these so-called idiopathic cases frequently depend upon some affection of the internal organs, they are, in point of fact, as true traumatic cases as any.

Although we cannot examine the irritated part with the eye during life, we have good reason for saying that the spinal chord itself is generally the part where the mischief commences; for if we irritate the spinal chord of an animal without pressure, we can cause tetanic spasms and symptoms (pressure produces palsy). Then, again, if the spinal chord of a frog be laid bare, and a drop of strychnine be applied, this will produce tetanic symptoms.

In speaking of strychnine producing tetanus, a German doctor administered nux vomica—which is the active principle of strychnine—to a number of patients, in all of which tetanic symptoms were observed whenever any cold draught assailed them. Again, tetanus is said to be a disease of the brain by some, but this is not the case. We are rather of opinion that it has its origin in that part of the spinal chord contained in the cranium, which is called the medulla oblongata, the spinal chord having a deal to do with regulating the motions of the body.

Then, again, in tetanus the brain has none of its functions impaired, such as hearing, seeing, smelling, tasting, &c. We have no reason, therefore, to conclude that the brain is diseased in consequence of this complaint. We must come to the conclusion that it is a disease of the medulla oblongata, because we can produce tetanic symptoms by applying irritation to that organ.

It is also said to be a disease of the voluntary

muscles; but I think it affects the involuntary ones also. We know how difficult it is to give an injection in this disease, owing to the constricted state of the sphincter ani; and we also know how difficult it is to get the bowels to open. This arises from the constricted state of the muscular coat of the intestines. The arterial tubes are also involved in the spasms, as they are now known to contain a certain quantity of involuntary muscular fibre, which is supplied by nerves.

The symptoms generally come on with a gradual accession, taking three or four days before they reach the worst stage. Should they get very severe by the second day, the patient seldom recovers, as the cases which reach their greatest intensity soonest are the worst to cure.

Tetanus may exist in all degrees of intensity; so much is this the case that even the thigh-bones in man are known to have been broken by it. This extraordinary rigidity of the muscles also causes the temperature to rise.

The first symptoms are a general stiffness of the loins, tucked-up belly, hardness of the muscles, and a slight erection of the tail; and in a day or two there is a visible stiffness of the jaws, accompanying which we have an abundant secretion of saliva. The head soon becomes drawn up by the rigidity of the muscles, then the membrane or cartilage of the eye drops down over the greater part of the ball; and when the head is suddenly elevated, this membrane will be seen protruded over the eye. As the disease becomes more aggravated, the hocks are turned out, the limbs stiff both before and behind, and the animal moves as if he were on stilts. The abdominal muscles are tucked up, and the muscles of respiration are rigid, causing difficulty in breathing. This also depends upon spasm of the muscles of the larynx. When the disease has attained this stage, the animal betrays great irritability if you approach him. The jaws are quite fixed, the membrane of the nose is reddened, while congestion of the lungs has set in. The nostrils are dilated, obstinate constipation is present, and the patient cannot urinate properly. This appears to be the only function in which secretion is not arrested, and he perspires copiously. The state of the pulse is remarkable in the first stage; it is generally *strong, but as the disease advances it becomes oppressed. We can feel a large artery, but no distinct beat. When an animal affected with tetanus lies down he seldom lives long, for he cannot breathe : therefore the longer he stands the longer he lives. Should an animal affected with this disease continue to live for a week or ten days, and by that time his bowels begin to act, he will, as a rule, pull through. But recovery is a slow process, and is always slowest in those cases in which the disease has been most acute, while some animals never recover thoroughly.

Causes.—We know that many cases arise from wounds, and we also know that irritation of the spinal chord will produce this disease: there is good reason to believe, therefore, that tetanus is caused by nervous or spinal irritation in every case. The majority of cases arise after wounds, but as to the exact time at which it does appear in our patients it is difficult to ascertain. All we know is, that it seems to come on just when the wound is healing, or perhaps has healed, and seems to result from a punctured wound rather than a lacerated one. It is a common notion that it follows wounds of the tendons, which belief has arisen from the fact that punctured wounds are generally below the knee and hock, in the legs or tendinous parts. The sudden action of a draught or cold air is very apt to hasten it.

The fatality in tetanus is great, for out of a hundred animals afflicted, from eighty to ninety will die.

Some people say that worms cause tetanus by producing derangement of the digestive system. All I can say is, that on making *post-mortem* examinations I have failed to trace it to such a cause.

It is a common disease in hot climates, and is said to destroy a greater number of black people than white.

Post-mortem Appearances.—These are somewhat variable, yet they show a certain degree of uniformity, for we always find intense congestion of the lungs, and from this we are bound to conclude that congestion accelerates death. On examining animals who have died of congestion, we often find them not so much congested as in cases of tetanus; therefore I think it fair and conclusive to assume that it accelerates death. This congestion seems to depend upon the confined action of the muscles of respiration. The spinal chord is also congested. It is a curious fact that the tetanic tension of the muscles disappears soon after death; but, of course, it will return in time, and then we have the hard firm feel of the muscles.

Again, rupture of the muscular fibres is frequently seen, consequently there is extravasation of blood. Sometimes several of the muscles are pale, the blood having been all squeezed out of them.

Foreign bodies have also been found in the wounds of tetanic patients. In some of these cases the irritation has been traced along the nerve to the spinal chord.

Treatment.—This disease has been, and still is, treated in all kinds of ways, and a very great deal has been said about it, as it is of such a serious nature. Those cases seem to do best in which we support the system, keeping the animal quiet and the bowels open. Earnest efforts to keep the bowels open by injections, &c., should be persevered in.

Among the innumerable remedies there is not one that has been so extensively used as opium, and many cases have recovered under the use of this drug. But when we consider the enormous quantity of opium an ox can take without producing any effect, particularly in this disease, one does not feel disposed to believe in the efficacy of it; for it is stated as a fact that in one case a man swallowed two ounces daily for eleven days in succession under tetanic spasms, and in the end died. There is another case on record, that of a man (he was a negro) who took one drachm every three hours for seventeen days. After taking this enormous quantity he recovered.

Abernethy once found thirty drachms of undissolved opium in the stomach of a tetanic patient who had died. Now, if we reflect upon the extraordinary quantity a man can take, and compare it with doses that are sometimes recommended for cattle, it compels one to question its efficacy.

When chloroform and ether were first found to possess a remarkable power of relieving spasms, it was thought they would prove of great benefit in this disease; and so they have in man, but as yet they have failed in cattle. I have administered chloroform on several occasions, in all of which it suspended the spasms for a time, but they always returned again. Many think that chloroform would be useful in mitigating the spasms in order to give other medicines; but although this allows us to open the jaws, these parties forget that it does not enable the animal to swallow. Many animals have been choked in this manner. Extract of belladonna is much used, and we must admit that many cases recover under it; therefore we are at times tempted to believe that it does possess a certain amount of utility. But we should examine both sides of the question, as in all cases I have seen of recovery from its use, I have found that the bowels were well opened before or during its action.

Again, extreme cold has been employed as a cure, for cold seems to relax the spasms; and animals have been plunged into cold water, or had it pumped over them. Sudden fright has also had the effect of relaxing the muscles; while eminent men in the profession recommend locking the door and putting the key in your pocket in order to secure absolute rest. But apart from all that, the best way is to get the bowels opened if possible, and afterwards give the belladonna; then allow the patient plenty of cool air. Keep him in a dark box, shutting out out all light, and leaving him in absolute quietness.

The next question is, What are we to do to keep up the system and the bowels open at the same time? The animal cannot take nourishment, as the mouth is closed; and even if open, he could not swallow it. In such a case gently elevate the head, then put a flexible tube down the nostrils, having a bladder fixed to the end of it containing either the medicines or gruel that you are about to administer;

then gently squeeze the bladder, allowing only a few drops to trickle down at first, which can be gradually increased as the patient gets used to it. Give also gruel-injections, which will be taken up into the system by absorption. Some people apply mercurial blisters along the spine, while others insert setons; but I think this is only adding irritation to irritation; therefore a good, fresh, newly-stripped sheepskin is the best and simplest thing to excite a copious action in the skin without producing irritation. Of course, unless the animal is a valuable one, it is perhaps as well to have it destroyed at once.

Chorea, or St. Vitus's Dance.

This disease is seen more frequently in the dog than in any other animal. It also occurs in children, and is seen occasionally in the horse and cow. The remarkable features of it consist in a combined or regular movement affecting certain groups of muscles, whose action is quite involuntary, and seems to be increased when the will is excited. It is apparently a disease of the spinal chord, affecting only the nerves of motion, and not those of sensation. This is proved by a man with chorea not having the spasms removed during sleep; for it has been demonstrated that the brain sleeps when men sleep, as is shown by tickling any one's foot while asleep; the sleeper will draw up his leg, but this is

H

done quite unconsciously. The symptoms are similar in all animals. Men stagger as though they were drunk, and look idiotic, though they are not. There is a continual twitching in the part that is affected, which is constantly in motion, either up and down or from side to side. Others, again, may appear all right when standing still, but immediately on attempting to lift the leg they find they cannot do it.

There is another form of chorea which comes on suddenly, and which it is well to guard against. If you go to put halters on some horses' heads, or look at their teeth, they will throw up their heads, fix their lips, and run backwards, the muscles of their necks becoming quite rigid.

Chorea may affect the head and neck only, or one leg; or the whole body may be affected, or only one-half; or sometimes the tail alone is implicated.

Again, a man afflicted with chorea, generally speaking, can run better than walk; just in the same way that a stammerer can sing better than talk.

In dogs it frequently follows distemper, but in the horse and cow we know not what it arises from.

There is no treatment available.

Megrims, Vertigo, or Giddiness.

This is sometimes, but improperly, called staggers, for it is only a symptom of the disease. The term "megrims" is of very common use in some parts of England, and seems to consist in a temporary loss of voluntary power and motion.

Symptoms.—The animal will often shake his head, thus showing the fit is coming on, then look at his flanks and fall down. There is no spasm while he lies on the ground, and hardly any pulse to be felt; but in a few minutes he will get up and give himself a shake, as if nothing had happened. This disease is frequently seen in farm-horses, particularly the heavy kind, and comes on while they are at work in the collar. This tends to convince me that it generally arises from temporary congestion of the brain, caused by obstruction of the jugular veins by the collar. Of course in cattle that are used for agricultural purposes a like result may be expected.

Treatment.—Allow the animal a roomy collar and food that will not constipate the bowels, giving an occasional dose of medicine.

Epilepsy, or Falling Sickness,

means "I seize"—"I seize upon." It is a cerebro-spinal disease, which may be idiopathic or symptomatic, spontaneous or accidental, and occurs in paroxysms, with uncertain intervals between each. These paroxysms are characterised by loss of consciousness, and by convulsive motions of the body. Frequently the fit comes on suddenly; at other times it is preceded by indisposition in the shape of indigestion, vertigo, or stupor.

At times, before the loss of consciousness occurs, a sensation as if of a cold vapour is detected. This appears to rise in one part of the body and proceed towards the head, when, as soon as it has reached the brain, the patient falls down. The ordinary duration of a fit is from five to twenty minutes; sometimes it goes off in a few seconds, at others it is protracted for hours. In all cases there is a loss of sensation, sudden falling down, distortion of the eyes and face, countenance of a red purple or violet colour, grinding of the teeth, foaming at the mouth, convulsions of the limbs, difficult respiration, at times stertorous, with sometimes an involuntary discharge of fæces and urine. When the fit has passed away, the patient seems not to recollect what has occurred for some time, and seems to be affected with headache, stupor, and lassitude.

The disease is cerebro-spinal, and is generally organic, but it may be functional and symptomatic of irritation in other parts, as in the stomach, bowels, &c., while the prognosis as to ultimate recovery is unfavourable. Epilepsy does not, however, frequently destroy life, but it is very apt to lead to mental prostration.

Post-mortem examinations have thrown no light upon the pathology of this malady.

During the attack of epilepsy the consciousness

of the patient becomes, in the mildest cases, completely lost; hence all the symptoms of the seizure cannot be described.

In the treatment of epilepsy the cause must be sought for, and if possible removed. During the paroxysms very little can be done, but as the tongue is then liable to be injured by the teeth, the jaws may be kept apart by putting a cork or piece of wood between them. If the fit has been brought on by indigestion, the offensive matters in the stomach must be cleared away. It is during the intervals that occur between the paroxysms that the greatest efforts must be made. Generally, there is considerable irritation and debility of the nervous system, hence tonics have been found the best remedies. Of these, perhaps, the most powerful in epilepsy is nitrate of silver, given regularly, and continued for months if necessary. Preparations of iron, copper, and zinc have also been used, with vegetable tonics, antispasmodics in general, counter-irritants, &c. Unfortunately, in many cases these remedies are found insufficient, consequently all that can be done is to palliate the disease by removing carefully the exciting causes, preventing strong emotions and violent exercise, and regulating the diet.

Hysteria.

This is an affection that only occurs in females. It generally assumes the form of paroxysms, the principal character of which consists in alternate fits of laughing and crying in the human subject, accompanied by a sensation as if a ball were ascending upwards towards the neck and producing strangulation. If the attack be violent there is sometimes loss of consciousness (although the presence of consciousness usually distinguishes hysteria frome epilepsy), with convulsions. The duration of the attack is very variable; it appears to be dependent upon irregularity of nervous distribution. During the fit, dashing cold water on the face, applying stimulants to the nose or given internally, and antispasmodics, form the principal curative agents.

Hydrocephalus, or Water in the Brain,

is generally seated, according to modern theories, in the meninges and surface of the encephalon. Its progress is extremely acute and often very rapid. It may be divided into three stages. The symptoms of the first stage are general febrile irritation and intolerance of light and sound, succeeded by delirium. Those of the second stage denote that the inflammation has ended in effusion, great slowness of pulse, moaning, and dilated pupils. In the third stage, profound stupor, paralysis, convulsions, involuntary evacuations, and quick pulse supervene, frequently accompanied by death.

The disease is of uncertain duration, sometimes destroying life in two or three days, in other cases extending over several weeks. If the prognosis is unfavourable, however, a dose of physic may be given, and a seton run through the skin at the top of the head.

DISEASES OF THE BLOOD.

The first is hyperæmia, which is a preternatural accumulation of blood in the capillary vessels, more especially local plethora or congestion. Various forms of blood-disease are admitted by pathologists; for example, the active or sthenic; the asthenic or passive; the cadaveric, or that which takes place immediately before or after death; the hypostatic, which occurs in depending parts; and the mechanical, which is produced by some impediment to the circulation.

The second is anæmia, loss of blood, or the opposite to plethora. It is characterised by signs of debility, with a diminished quantity of fluids in the capillary vessels. The essential character of the blood in this disease is diminution in the quantity of red corpuscles.

Third, leucocythæmia, a condition of the blood which consists in a superabundant development of white corpuscles. This is a disease which has been observed at times to be accompanied by enlargement of the spleen and liver.

Fourth, pyæmia, a purulent contamination of the blood, producing marked depression of the vital powers, and the formation of abscesses in various regions of the body. It is supposed by some to be due to suppurative capillary phlebitis, by others to coagulation of the vitiated blood in the vessels—especially the veins—or the heart, and to the inflammation and suppuration developed by the clots of blood when detached and carried into the capillaries of other parts.

Fifth, glycohæmia, which indicates a saccharine condition of the blood.

Sixth, uræmia, a condition of the blood in which it contains, or is presumed to contain, urea, and to give rise to sundry morbid phenomena implicating the nervous centres more especially.

Seventh, acholia, a deficiency or want of bile.

Eighth, piarhæmia, or fat in the blood.

Erysipelas

is a disease of frequent occurrence in man, and a peculiar one it is. The inflammation which accompanies it is of a very singular character in man as well as in the horse. It is an inflammatory disease affecting the submucous tissue or the surface of mucous cavities, and is identified by various names, such as the "rose" and "St. Anthony's fire." The inflammation is peculiar for running into rapid exudation, is strikingly indisposed to the formation of pus, but greatly given to sloughing. It is very common in the horse, but is of more frequent occurrence in the cow.

When it does occur, it may exist independently, or coexist with other diseases. When independent, it seems generally to come on without any assignable cause, but in the majority of instances it follows the same course as diseases of a debilitating nature. It seems also to depend upon a difference in the circulating fluid. The fibrin in this case is increased, yet the exudation does not seem to form pus.

Symptoms.—It generally begins below and extends upwards; but it may commence in any part of the body—usually the legs or head. Wherever it originates the skin is thickened and raised up, and feels brawny, like the skin of swine—that is, hard, rough, and rigid. This is distinguished from the swelling of purpura by always being red from the beginning, does not pit on pressure, while there is an abrupt line between the healthy and diseased parts. Even the very hair feels rougher and harder, and if you touch the skin it causes intense pain.

I have seen cases where the heads of the patients were so heavy that they could not lift them up, and the same may be said of the legs. The pulse will be quick, breathing hurried, considerable fever present, and appetite suspended.

This condition of swelling may affect one or all the legs at once, or the head only. These swellings have the appearance as if you had tied a cord tight round the limb to prevent circulation.

Treatment.—It is very important to have the bowels opened in this disease, which can be accomplished by the diet. With reference to medicines, I must recommend diuretics and vegetable tonics. If the season admit, give green food. This acts beneficially upon the bowels, and with them and the kidneys in motion the patient will soon pull through. The local treatment consists in hot applications, and the liberal use of lard or oil to the swollen parts. Should the disease extend in spite of all you can do, incisions should be made, about two or three inches long, between the healthy and the diseased parts.

Black Quarter, Quarter Ill, Black Leg, or Splenic Apoplexy.

This disease attacks young growing cattle, and is attended with startling fatality. It is a congestive form of putrid fever, due to a morbid state of the blood and congestive state of the system. It may be characterised as a true blood-disease of a reducing and typhoid nature. It is specially due to a deficiency of fibrin, and as a result of this the blood loses its coagulability, while the red corpuscles are in a disintegrated state.

Some cattle are more susceptible to this disease than others, especially young, growing, well-bred animals. Calves have been known to take this disease when about three months old. All animals that recover have only been externally affected.

Symptoms.—These appear very suddenly. The stock may be inspected at night, and to all appearance every one is improving in a satisfactory way; in the morning, however, one may be found dead or dying. At first there is great fever, which gradually increases without the least intermission; the mouth is hot and dry; the pulse quick, with irregular beat; the animal is frequently unconscious, and when moved does so with a staggering gait, with accompanying lameness in one or more limbs. The swelling must be attentively watched, which occurs in either the breast, neck, or quarters, and cannot well be mistaken, as it has a crepitating or crackling sound. This is an important symptom, and one that ought to be borne in mind. The urine is scanty and high-coloured; the animal froths at the mouth; eyes staring and bloodshot; the breathing becomes very rapid, and the animal drops down dead.

Treatment.—This is a matter of considerable difficulty. Owing to the rapidity of the disease there is little or no time for treating it. If only one is affected, give a purge immediately, and keep the patient walking about. At the same time take prompt measures to arrest the further progress of the disease. This can be accomplished by inserting a seton through the dewlap, which is a very simple but most effectual preventive, as it increases the deficient element in the blood, fibrin. This must be followed up by alterative medicine and a complete change of diet. Allow the seton to remain in for three weeks, then remove.

Post-mortem Appearances.—Some writers endeavour to classify and separate black quarter from splenic apoplexy, but there is in reality very little difference between the two diseases, therefore I have described them conjointly.

The blood is thin and watery; does not coagulate, but passes readily into a state of putrefaction. Should a dog or cat partake of a portion of the diseased meat in a raw state, it will soon terminate its existence. The spleen is sometimes ruptured, and always engorged with dark blood, and is often twice its natural size. The lungs are also sometimes soft and enlarged, and the small intestines in an inflammatory condition; but the removal of the skin is sufficient to show the cause of death, for it will be found covered with patches. Strict precaution ought to be observed in regard to the man that is employed to do this work, for should he have a scratch or cut upon his hand, it will in all likelihood lead to blood-poisoning, which may terminate fatally.

Glossanthrax, or Carbuncle of the Tongue.

This is another blood-disease, and affects the mucous membrane of the mouth and tongue. It is of a low typhoid nature, preceded by passive congestion; it occurs often as an epizootic, and is met with in full-grown cattle.

Symptoms are, great fever; difficulty in breathing; mouth open; tongue swollen and protruded beyond the lips; swelling of the face; saliva dribbling from the mouth, which becomes thicker as the disease advances, and in bad cases is mixed with blood; watery secretion from the nose and eyes; the tongue partakes of a livid hue, and sometimes becomes gangrenous, whitish vesicles appearing over its surface, with a dark rim surrounding them. As a rule, it is accompanied by diarrhœa, and the patient commonly dies from apnœa.

Treatment.—Freely scarify the parts affected; open the carbuncle; wash out the mouth with a weak solution or astringent, such as alum; give a mild laxative, followed up with tonics and good food, which must be soft in order that the patient may be enabled to masticate it.

Aphtha, or Thrush.

This consists of roundish, pearl-coloured vesicles, confined to the lips, mouth, and intestinal canal, and generally terminates in curd-like sloughs.

Symptoms.—Swelling of the membrane that lines the mouth, the lips having an elevated appearance when the animal's mouth is shut.

Treatment.—Give a dose of purgative medicine,

wash out the mouth with astringent solutions, and give sloppy food. If the animal be weak and in low condition, give tonics and stimulants, with cold water to drink, in which may be dissolved a little nitre.

Composition of the Bones.

Before entering on the diseases that are peculiar to bones, it will be advantageous to the reader to understand the structure and composition of the material that supports the weight of the animal and protects the internal organs.

Bone is composed of two distinct parts—namely, earthy and animal matter—in the following proportions:—

Phosphate of lime,	51.04
Chloride of lime,	2.00
Soda and chloride of sodium,	1.20
Carbonate of lime,	11.30
Carbonate of magnesia,	1.16
Gelatine and fat,	33.30
Total,	100.00

The earthy and animal matters are so completely blended together that they appear like a homogeneous mass. Such, however, is not the case, as they can be separated in the following manner:— If you steep a bone in hydrochloric acid, you can dissolve out the earthy matter; and by burning, you leave the earthy matter, while you destroy the animal matter. These earthy salts are found in all animal structures. If a transverse section is made in a bone, thus ▭, an opening will be found called the haversian canal, which ramifies into the compact structure. Around these canals the osseous matter is deposited in layers or laminæ. Surrounding these canals are spaces of an oval shape, termed lacunæ, or empty spaces. There are also numerous fine thread-like canals which run outwards from the haversian ones, and, joining the lacunæ, are termed canaliculi, or little canals. Inside of these are the true bone-cells, extending from the lacunæ to the haversian canal, which conveys the plasma of the blood, thereby affording nourishment to the whole bone.

Bones are covered with a material called periosteum, which is composed of fibrous tissue adhering firmly to the bone. This periosteum is the chief source of supply for the compact tissue. It is from its inner surface that the blood-vessels pass into the cancellated tissue. The bone also receives support from the nutrient arteries which traverse the internal canal, and then break up into fine plexuses of blood-vessels.

DISEASES OF THE BONE.

Rachitis.

When bones are deficient in earthy matter, we generally find rachitis present. In this disease the bones are imperfectly ossified. It occurs in two forms, acute and chronic. Young animals are liable to attacks of the acute form, known as joint-ill. It affects the articulations, causing lameness with swelling of the joints, more especially those of the knee. The inflammation increases, so does the lameness; suppuration sets in, and the result is open joints. This form of the disease terminates fatally, as the patient wastes away, and ultimately dies in great agony.

Causes.—Insufficient supply of milk and exposure to damp and cold; also where the water that is used is soft and deficient in lime salts, one of the essential constituents of bone.

Treatment.— As the causes are removable, strict attention must be paid to them. With careful management the disease may be avoided, and its prevention is easier and better than cure.

In the chronic or subacute form, the shaft of the bone towards its extremities begins to bend. This will not happen until the animal is six or eight months old. Therefore commence at once by giving an excess of lime-water, with small quantities of good linseed-cake; in fact, the best food and shelter at command. Put splints on the limb and bandage up, but not too tight, when it will again recover something like its former shape.

Mollities Ossium

occurs in full-grown animals, but presents no symptoms during life. It is a constitutional disease, being the conversion of the animal bases into fat; such subjects are liable to exostosis. There is no treatment available.

Osteo-Porosis.

In this disease there is a distension of the haversian canals, which contain a juicy fluid, along with the blood-vessels. It is seen when the distension is most active, the parts being in a highly vascular condition. Professor Williams thinks it is owing to a deficiency in the material for building up the haversian canals, consequently the blood-vessels force themselves in, and the walls distend.

Symptoms.—Swelling of the face and discharge from nostrils, the patient being unable to masticate its food. This disease, the same authority says, arises from outward causes; but if we have a discharge from the nose, it may be due to derangement of the

I

fifth nerve, which nerve seems to preside over the nutrition of the face.

Treatment.—Unsatisfactory.

Osteo-Sarcoma, or Fleshy and Bone Tumour,

frequently affects cattle, and attacks the jaws. It has no connection with the teeth, as supposed by some. In nasal gleet we may find such a tumour, which must be removed by the knife.

Enchondroma, or Tumour on the Sternum or Chest.

This tumour may be hard, hot, and painful to the touch, and if allowed to continue, becomes converted into cartilage and fibrous tissue.

Caries and Necrosis of Bone.

There is not an extremity of the bones which is not liable to caries. This disease corresponds to ulcer of the soft parts; in its course it is frequently chronic, although from the devastation it produces (especially in the true hock-joint), it appears to be acute.

When caries is superficial, it presents the appearance of a moth-eaten substance. When it affects a large articulation, accompanied with bleeding, it is both a diagnostic and fatal sign, because the laminar layer has been removed; hence the haversian canals and blood-vessels are now exposed to the friction of the part.

The discharge from a carious bone is of an acrid nature, and will blacken a silver probe. Caries is healed by a change of unhealthy to healthy granulations.

Treatment, to be successful, depends greatly upon subduing the inflammation. If in an open joint, the application of a counter-irritant will assist in its prevention.

Necrosis

is in every way analogous to mortification of a soft structure, and differs from caries by the vitality of the part being entirely destroyed. It resembles dry gangrene, and arises from some external injury to the bone, or from any cause by which the bone is laid bare or crushed.

Necrosis is of two kinds, total and partial. The boundaries of a necrosed bone are irregular in every way. It produces extensive inflammation in the adjoining healthy bone and tissue. Suppuration takes place, and goes on until the offending portion or necrosed part of the bone is removed. The pus discharges itself externally, carrying with it small pieces of the diseased bone. It is distinguished by its bleached appearance and irregular borders. The bone in contact with it assumes a rosy colour, becomes succulent, and is finally removed by absorption. The line dividing the two is called the line of demarcation.

The inflammation that exists leads to a deposit being thrown out beneath the periosteum; and as this extends into the interior, the bony matter is there deposited. Causes are intrinsic and extrinsic: in the former no remedy can be suggested; in the latter, remove the bone, giving tonics, good food, and lime-water to drink.

TUMOURS.

This department is well represented in the human subject, and unfortunately they appear in all shapes, sizes, and situations; but in veterinary practice we find them much less numerous, and in general not of a very malignant character.

Tumours may be defined to be perceptible or definite additions to the substance of any part of the body. They occur under two principal characters: First, there is a class of tumours made up of textures similar to those already existing in the body, such as bones, cartilage, &c. These are called non-malignant tumours, and are by far the most numerous kind met with in our practice. Secondly, there are tumours composed of tissue not existing naturally in the body, and which have a tendency to destroy and poison the body, hence they are called malignant or destructive tumours. This class, however, is very rare; we cannot, however, always draw a definite line between the two, although there is no doubt that some tumours begin non-malignant, and then assume a malignant type.

Non-malignant Tumours.—These are composed, as I have said, of materials already existing in the body, such as cartilage and bone, becoming enlarged, without any structural difference. The character of a non-malignant tumour is that it does not destroy, poison, or spread to surrounding tissues, having no tendency to reproduction, and when thoroughly removed the animal recovers. Tumours of this description seldom run on to suppuration or ulceration, yet they may destroy life; but this is not due to poisoning of the system, but from their mechanical inconvenience.

Malignant Tumours, on the other hand, such as cancer, always do destroy, change, and alter the textures surrounding them into their own textures, while they poison the whole system, and are apt to grow faster than non-malignant ones. They are often connected with constitutional disorder, frequently running on to softening and ulceration.

These tumours cause pain and intense irritation in their neighbourhood, and when removed, there is no guarantee that they will not be reproduced in the same or another site. In one sense they are not themselves a local disease, but rather indications of a disease which has a constitutional seat or origin.

It is a remarkable and admitted fact that people

with tumours will live longer without having them removed than those that have them cut away. At the same time the formation of tumours is very much influenced by the constitution of the animal; and this is the case in cattle as well as in the horse. In bitches, again, it often assumes a hereditary character, and what causes it in one will not do so in another. Thus a human subject may receive an injury on the breast, and get well again without much trouble; whereas another may receive a similar injury, and, particularly if there is any constitutional diathesis, a tumour may be the result.

Horses are not so liable to tumours as cows, and cows are not so liable as bitches, for in the latter animals we have them almost as frequently as in mares.

The chemical constituents of tumours vary. The proximate principles which are chiefly formed in them are fat, gelatine, and albumen, and according as any of these predominate in the structure, the nature of the tumour is found to alter. It is a circumstance to be noted that the malignant tumours contain a great amount of albumen with fat, while non-malignant ones consist principally of gelatine.

The great majority of tumours are enclosed in a cavity called a sac, especially those of a non-malignant nature; but tumours in the brain are not usually invested with a wall. On the other hand, a malignant tumour is seldom enclosed in a cyst, so that it is difficult to say where the healthy texture begins and the unhealthy ends ; whereas, in the non-malignant, we have a pretty definite line of demarcation.

Malignant tumours in cattle are situated most commonly at the root of the tongue and in the eyes, affecting the orbits, also the glands of the neck and the external organs of generation. From this it may be seen that they are rather inclined to affect the same situations in cattle as they do in women. They are classified under the general term of cancers, of which there are various kinds, known, first, by the name of *medullary*, so called because they resemble the medullary substance of the brain ; second, *scirrhous*, or hard cancer, which is always painful ; third, *colloid*, or glue-like cancer—but this kind is never seen in the lower animals ; fourth, *fungus hæmatodes*, or bleeding cancer.

The scirrhous kind occurs most commonly in the udders of the cow and bitch, and the lips of the external organs of generation.

In the bitch it seems to come on without any apparent cause, and is slow in growth, but gradually increases to an enormous size, causing great pain and inconvenience. One feature which distinguishes scirrhous from any other tumour is that it seems to involve the skin. It is also red, and appears to be attached to the surrounding tissues, and soon ulcerates. If the skin is loose, can be easily moved from the tumour, and does not appear to affect the surrounding tissues, but is hard and knotty, we may be satisfied that it is not a cancerous tumour. When we examine the tumour, there is generally found one opening, and sometimes more, leading into it. These orifices have a ring of proud flesh round their margins, and if you cut into them with a knife, they are always hard, and resist like cartilage. When examined under the microscope, the tumour is found to be composed of fibrous tissue. Its base is enclosed, in which are cells, thus showing that it belongs to the malignant class. These cells are large, containing other cells or nuclei having the power of reproduction; and, in addition, there is a kind of granular juicy matter by which the cells are nourished. Therefore, owing to the presence of these cells we must look upon the tumour as of a malignant character. Medullary tumours are found in the head, glands of the neck, and liver, and contain the same cells as the scirrhous kind, but in greater proportion, with less fibrous tissue. They are known by their vascularity, by their adhering to the parts in which they exist, and from certain orifices leading to them, which are also surrounded by a ring of proud flesh.

Fungus hæmatodes are those which contain a great amount of blood-vessels and cells, with scarcely any fibrous tissue. This sort of tumour grows more rapidly than any of the others. They bleed profusely on the slightest touch; and if you cut them away they grow again, and are very unsatisfactory to deal with.

Non-Malignant Tumours

are more common to the lower animals than the malignant kind. Sometimes they are of enormous size and weight, and generally occur about the anus or generative organs. In the horse they are not of a malignant type, but are regarded so in man, as they generally occur in combination with cancer. Warts will sometimes grow to a great size, and frequently appear again after being cut away. This is not owing to their being malignant, but to the difficulty of removing the roots thoroughly

A polypus is a kind of pendulous growth, generally attached to some superficial mucous membrane, and is found most frequently in the nose, larynx, vagina, and sometimes at the entrance to the uterus. It usually consists of a thickening of the mucous membrane. When it occurs in the nose, it assumes a variety of shapes, but the most common is usually that of a pear, with a bulb and neck.

Symptoms.—If in the nose, there is difficulty in breathing, accompanied with a kind of snore, particularly in inspiration; and if situated far back, there will be a tendency to suffocation. We can generally see the polypi, and they must be cut or twisted away.

138   DISEASES OF CATTLE.

Warts comprise several kinds, but they are of two chief characters in the lower animals. They are either on the surface, or just underneath the skin. The former is called the common or epidermic wart; the latter the fibrous, cystic, or subcutaneous wart.

Epidermic or common warts are well known to all, especially in the human subject; they also appear upon the skin of horses and cattle. There is no essential structural difference between the one and the other, though in cattle we find them much rougher on the surface than in the human being. In warts both layers of the skin are involved; namely, the epidermis or cuticle, which consists of scales similar to the scales of a fish, though not so large; it is not vascular, and contains no blood-vessels or nerves. Underneath is the true skin (cutis vera), which consists of blood-vessels, fibrous tissue, and nerves.

In the horse, these warts are frequently seen about the nostrils, eyelids, face, sheath, and between the fore and hind legs; and in cattle they occur chiefly under the abdomen and on the teats and sides of the face; indeed, all parts of the skin are subject to them; but some breeds of horses and cattle are more liable to warts than others. They are of two varieties—one of them shooting up perpendicularly or abruptly, the other merely spreading along the surface in patches. This does not depend upon any difference in their structure, but in their development, the single ones having generally a well-defined neck, especially when of large size.

Warts always first occur in a small pimple, and when large they are very vascular. They are more common in young animals of all kinds than in old ones, therefore I think that their occurrence is owing to some irregular growth of the skin. If we take a slice of the rough surface and examine it under the microscope after having placed it in acetic acid, we find it made up of little cells, inside of which smaller ones are found; and in proportion to the size of the wart, so is the size of the vessels involved.

Treatment.—All kinds of charms were had recourse to at one time to banish warts, but of course no one entertains these superstitious ideas now. Sometimes they will disappear of themselves, but the treatment must vary according to the kind of warts you encounter. If you find a wart with a broad fleshy base, hard, and not large, you had better cut it away at once. Apply the actual cautery, or some strong caustic, so as to destroy the growing surface. Of the two I prefer the hot iron. Should the wart have a neck, you can tie a string round sufficiently tight to arrest its supply of blood, when it will die and slough off. In this case it is always better to apply the cautery after the wart has dropped off, in order to destroy any remaining root.

When warts occur over the surface of the skin

you should cut away all the horny parts, wipe off the blood, and apply caustics or the hot iron. In some cases you have to repeat the cutting, so as to allow the caustic to penetrate deep enough. Cattle are very liable to have them on their tails. In these cases cut the warts away and apply the hot iron.

There is another kind somewhat common in cattle, called fibrous or subcutaneous cystic warts. These may vary in size from a marble to a 20-lb. weight. They do not involve the skin, for you can move it over their surface in any way you choose, which shows that they are not connected with the muscles. There is no pain on pressure unless the skin is ulcerated—which is the case sometimes—and there is no sensible increase of heat. They are hard, and move readily. The tissues below the skin do not become ulcerated owing to the non-malignity of the wart, but simply to the mechanical inconvenience it causes; for if we cut the skin away, we come to a great amount of fibrous tissue into which numerous blood-vessels ramify, and from which the sac or wall receives its nutrition and growth. Inside this sac is the proper wart, consisting of a dense mass of inorganic matter: it is very rare that there are any blood-vessels in it.

When these warts are small it is very easy removing them, by making a single incision through the skin and squeezing them out. A good-sized wart may be removed in this way. When you have a large one, and the skin ulcerated, it is more difficult to remove; therefore you must make two incisions similar to straight lines and get to the bottom of the sac or wall. It is from this wall the wart forms, so it must be removed.

Occasionally in cattle, though not so often as in man, we find fibrous tumours affecting the internal organs, such as the kidneys, uterus, &c., but most commonly on the inside of the cheeks, particularly of dogs; in this case they can be removed.

There is another kind of tumour occurring behind the elbow in cattle, of a fibrous nature, formed from the lymph; this is caused by the animal bruising that part in lying down on its heels. If the cause is not prevented, inflammation of a slow form takes place, and lymph is formed, with the result that a tumour is produced. In such a case blisters do no good; the warts ought to be cut out.

Fatty Tumours

are very rare in any of the lower animals, but there is a kind of tumour that forms on the backs of horses, under the saddle, also on the shoulder and under the collar, very much resembling fatty tumours, which is composed of fibrous tissue and fat.

Calcareous Tumours

(so named because they consist of inorganic matter) are generally called bony tumours, though they are not true bone, as they contain neither haversian canals, lacunæ, or canaliculi, but consist chiefly of the phosphates and carbonates of lime. These tumours may be found attached to the parts in which they are formed, as in tendons; or unattached, as in the skin. When they are in the latter, the hair falls off in patches, while the whole coat has a general unthriftiness about it.

Treatment.—The best remedy is to cut the tumours out. Sometimes they are found in the udders of bitches, where they arrest the flow of milk. The brain, also, is said to become ossified, but this is not the case; simple carbonates and phosphates have been deposited between the interstices of that organ, thus leading to the deception. The heart, surface of the lungs, testicles, &c., are also subject to the same disease.

Encysted Tumours

are those in which the contents are fluid instead of solid. This fluid is contained in a bag, which is likewise enclosed in an outer cyst or sac. These tumours are not frequently found in our patients, but when they do occur, they are generally found at the back part of the tongue. There seems to be no doubt about the origin of many of them; namely, that they are nothing more than a dilated follicle of a gland, arising from some obstruction. When they occur on the tongue, the obstruction may be a foreign body getting into the follicle, such as a hayseed, thus causing irritation to set in on the edges of the follicle. Lymph is exuded, and in time the orifice is plugged up; consequently dilatation of the follicle takes place, owing to an accumulation of its contents, which are found to consist of a cheesy fluid. They are distinguishable from a fibrous tumour by their elasticity, and they can be easily removed. There is nothing malignant about them; but when they do cause death, it arises from mechanical inconvenience, for in the larynx these tumours produce suffocation, and in the nose difficulty of breathing. In some parts of England this disease is very common.

Treatment.—When they occur on the tongue, and you can reach them, clip them off; and if upon any external surface, cut them out.

Cartilaginous or Enchondromatis Tumours

are very common in man, but in our patients we find them of rare occurrence. They do not often ulcerate; but when they are situated on parts where you can get at them, remove them. Once thoroughly removed, they seldom grow again.

Melanotic Tumours

occur frequently in the horse, but seldom in the cow. They differ in every way from other tumours, being composed of a black colouring matter, similar to charcoal, that is infiltrated into the tissues of the part on which they form. These tumours are most common in bright-grey and white horses, but are rare in dark-coloured animals. They are found oftenest in those places where the skin is tinged with black—such as the nose, eyelids, lips, sheaths, anus, lips of the vagina, and inside the legs, these parts not being covered with hair. Here it is important to inquire why they occur in white horses, and why in the dark part of the skin? These are questions not easily answered, although I think we can partially account for the phenomena. For instance, in a black horse the whole skin is equally covered by the black colouring matter called pigment; the same peculiarity characterises the bay or chesnut; consequently these tumours depend upon the presence of this pigment. In a white horse, the skin and hair are devoid of this pigment, yet he contains in his blood the materials for its formation; therefore it is reasonable to suppose that the body, being white, possesses no power to cause this matter to settle elsewhere than upon the dark places mentioned, where it is deposited in undue quantities.

When we examine its structure, we find the pigment consists of minute crystals. These are not enclosed in sacs, but graduate insensibly into the healthy parts, so that you cannot tell where the one begins and the other ends; while they depend upon the infiltration of the pigment into the tissues, to add to their bulk. This pigment also consists of iron and sulphur in great proportion. These tumours are not malignant in the lower animals, but are considered so in man, as in him they are frequently combined with cancer. There is a law in surgery that one should save as much skin as possible in operating, so as to cover up the wound with it, provided it is not diseased; but in this case we are compelled to cut a great deal of skin away, in consequence of its being diseased. In cases where the tumour has grown within the anus, it cannot be dissected out very well; but we need not fear making a cut into it. A good deal of bleeding may be caused, but when the vessels are properly secured the surface will soon heal; this will prove that it is not malignant. Still they should not be interfered with, unless you can remove them entirely, as they will, in most cases, grow again.

Scrofulous Tumours.

This disease is sometimes seen in the horse, though not often; it is more common in cattle, and still more so in the dog, but most of all in swine. In London about 1000 people die weekly, and out of this number 120 fall under this scrofulous diathesis.

Symptoms.—In the human subject there is a fair skin, large eyes, large lymphatic glands, especially about the neck, and large veins. In cattle the glands about the neck are the most liable to be attacked; in such cases we often have very large swellings. Young cattle are more subject to these collections of matter than old ones, particularly those that have come from inland counties, and are afterwards located near the sea-coast. Clyers is the name given to these swellings in England; and farms that are exposed to east winds, near the sea, and situate in low-lying damp localities, are most likely to be affected by them.

The characteristics of these tumours are—they are hard, deeply seated, involving the glands of the neck and angle of the jaws, and do not move under the skin as some tumours, which shows that they are in the tissues, so you cannot tell where they end. Sometimes they ulcerate; and when this takes place there is no longer any doubt about the nature of them.

Treatment.—Some cut them out, but this is not to be recommended, as it cannot be done without great loss of blood, owing to so many blood-vessels being in the part. The best thing to do is to shelter the animals well from wet and cold, make them otherwise comfortable, and by good feeding get them ready for the butcher as quickly as possible.

DISEASES OF THE SKIN, Etc.

The skin is that material which covers the body, and is an organ which performs the operations of absorption and secretion. It contains hair-follicles and two distinct sets of glands, namely, the sudoriferous or true sweat-glands, which are composed of coiled tubes; and the sebaceous, which secrete an oily fluid. These are found under the true skin, and the ducts of these glands are found opening into the hair-follicles.

The skin is subject to congestion, dropsy, inflammation, new formations (such as warts, &c.), and parasitic diseases.

Congestion is characteristic of low diseases, and may arise from mechanical obstruction. When it is very intense it gives rise to hæmorrhage into the subcutaneous tissue.

Dropsy is a result of congestion, and is easily defined in patients with swelled legs.

Inflammation may be either superficial or deep seated. Good examples of this are furnished in frosty weather by cracked heels, &c.; the animals move stiffly on their legs, and the skin is very painful to the touch.

Treatment.—Applications of warm water, applying ol. oliva two parts, liq. plumbi dia. one part, twice a day to irritated portions of the skin.

Ringworm.

This is a frequent disease in cattle. It generally makes its appearance about the eyelids. The hair commences to fall off; by degrees the disease extends all round and continues to spread, a kind of watery scales appearing. It occurs mostly in young animals, especially calves; in which it has occasionally been so much developed as to destroy numbers at a time.

Treatment.—Acetic acid. A few applications of this will cure it; or iodine one drachm, lard one ounce, mixed and applied; and in bad cases the iodide of silver may be adopted.

Wounds

are of five kinds: 1st, incised; 2d, punctured; 3d, contused; 4th, lacerated; 5th, gunshot.

1st, The *Incised* wound is made with a clean-cutting instrument, and is a clean smooth cut through the skin and connective tissue.

Treatment. — Arrest the bleeding, if any, and remove irritants.

Professor Syme taught that the parts should be left open and not brought together until six hours after, or till the serous discharge ceases to flow, when the wound will be found glazed over. This is due to a coating of fibrin, and if united now the edges readily adhere. Afterwards keep the animal quiet and dress with the following : Liq. plumbi dia. two drachms, zinc sulp. two drachms, water eight ounces. Mix this and apply night and morning.

2d, A *Punctured* wound is the most dangerous of all, as from its depth it is apt to implicate arteries, veins, nerves, and deep-seated vital parts. The parts traversed are often stretched and torn, and are liable to inflammation and suppuration. Pus forms, and, having no free exit, burrows under the surrounding tissue. Then, again, foreign bodies are liable to be carried into the wound to a great depth, and are never suspected until inflammation has set in. Wounds of this class are very apt to produce tetanus or locked-jaw.

Treatment.—Dilate and enlarge the wounds (this holds good in every case in the horse) so as to allow a free exit to matter or pus. The pus formed in a punctured wound carries off the dead tissue found in the part. If the pain is great and fever present, give a dose of physic to open the bowels, with opium and aconite to allay the pain and fever, and keep the animal upon soft sloppy food. Wounds of this description heal from the bottom towards the surface ; but if you suspect any hollow, open up the wound again and allow it to heal properly. It is a bad plan to probe a wound if it is near a joint, as it sets up suppuration.

3d, The third class may be placed under two heads ; *Contused* and *Ecchymosed*. This kind is produced by a blunt instrument causing injury with no laceration of the skin, when it is termed ecchymosis—a familiar example of which is to be seen in a man having a black eye. In this case there is, first, a benumbing of the parts, and then structural inflammation arises, the degree of which greatly depends upon the force of the blow.

4th, *Lacerated.* — This kind is attended with more hæmorrhage than an incised wound; but, the surfaces being irregular and ragged, the blood effused adheres; and so, if the arteries are torn, they consequently heal quicker than when cut.

Treatment.—Bleeding to be restrained, and all irritants removed; while the parts must be brought together, and quietness enjoined. In laceration of the lips, the depending parts should not be cut off, but well cleaned and brought together, when the wound may heal nicely, leaving a smaller scar than if you had employed the knife. When the fever is subdued, give good food in order that the blood may be supplied with the requisite material for the repair of these parts.

Open Joints.

In the treatment of open joints, let it ever be remembered that upon no consideration must one be induced or tempted to remove the coagulation, as it prevents the air from entering the cavity and causing irritation. If it is possible to stop up the wound at once, you should make it your endeavour to do so; but if the case has gone on for a day or so, pus will be formed and must have exit, so plugging will not do then. You must employ fomentations at first, to be followed by the application of a smart blister, which is an invaluable remedy. In this case the blister acts in three ways:—first, by producing swelling, which closes up the wound more or less; second, by keeping the animal quiet; third, by setting up the process of repair within the part.

During the progress of open joints you will see small abscesses forming, which burst and discharge synovia. Do not open these, but allow them to burst of themselves. Long rest is generally required before you can succeed in these cases; therefore, unless the animal is for breeding purposes, it had better be slaughtered at once.

Burns and Scalds

are divided into three classes, namely, burns producing redness, with loss of hair; burns producing vesicles, or blisters; and burns producing sloughing, or mortification of the parts. For those producing only a slight redness of the skin, paint the parts with a camel-hair brush dipped in a solution of nitrate of silver, five grains to one ounce of water, and after one coat has dried put on another; secondly, those attended by a degree of inflammation—producing vesicles in abundance, which sometimes turn into obstinate ulcers—should be treated with limewater and linseed-oil, or a solution of the nitrate of silver.

Constitutional Symptoms present.—The pulse weak; the animal shivers all over, blows, and is very much depressed. These symptoms must be overcome by giving stimulants and opium to relieve the pain. In some cases, where you have an extensive burn with the skin destroyed, the parts slough to a great extent, leaving underneath a texture of a pale-yellowish colour, very difficult to heal.

Treatment.—Subdue the fever by giving a laxative and aconite, then paint over the surface a solution of nitrate of silver. After a day or so the surrounding parts will swell; a line of demarcation will then present itself between the healthy and unhealthy parts; and where pus is formed, you should foment the parts with warm water, and dress with oil and limewater, or opium and oil. Afterwards, when the granulations become healthy, apply astringents.

Repair of Tissue.

The power of reproduction is certainly remarkable in the lower class of animals; but in those we have to deal with this power is limited to three classes of tissues—viz., first, those reproduced by nutrition and repetition, such as blood and epithelium; second, those of the lowest organisation and lowest chemical composition, such as gelatine, bones, &c.; third, those inserted into other tissues, not, however, essential to their structure.

Epithelium, when stripped of the mucous membrane, is reproduced as well as in nerve fibres; but the other tissues are only liable to repair, their place being taken by a low form of organised tissue. Dr. Hunter says: " When a wound has no external communication with the atmosphere, it rarely inflames, or only to a slight extent; but if exposed, it will both inflame and suppurate."

Healing of Wounds

takes place in four different ways—namely, by primary adhesion, granulation, secondary adhesion, and healing under a scab.

Dr. Hunter again says "that union by the first intention is caused by a fibrous exudate being thrown out, glueing the lips together and becoming organised, thus joining the parts." Blood extravasated is therefore not without its influence on the healing of wounds, although it is not required for the healing by the first intention. Again, if blood is left in a wound it is apt to produce inflammation; therefore it ought to be removed, as in some instances it becomes organised. The best time to remove a clot of blood is the second or third day.

The new material for repair is generally called

coagulable lymph; and this lymph is composed of fibrin, a little fatty matter, and a few saline constituents. It may be designated a living fluid, as it possesses the vital power of developing itself from inherent elements contained within, and is classified with fluids that have the property of assuming organised structure, which, as said before, exist in itself.

The principal material for the repair of wounds is lymph, which has a tendency to develop into fibrous or areolar tissue; but in some cases it deviates from this line, as in the case of fractures, where it may proceed at once to fibro-cartilage, which may become ossified. The lymph develops itself into areolar tissue from nucleated cells, these cells containing nucleoli, which are filled with granules. After a time they elongate. These processes are seen coming from the extremities, which form into a fibre, one cell after another going through the same process. In this way fibrous tissue is developed.

Primary adhesion is accomplished in the following manner: when the divided edges are allowed to remain open till the mouths of the vessels are closed, inflammation is set up, lymph is thrown out, and the edges are united.

Granulation.—When a wound fails to heal by the first intention, it then heals by granulation; blood gradually ceases to flow from the wound, and a whitish film collects over the surface, which is found to contain a number of corpuscles, and these become adhesive. If the wound remain open, the fibrin collects, while there is in and about it a period of inaction, the blood during that time becoming stagnant, or nearly so; hence materials cannot be given off for repair. Again, in healthy repair the blood is rapid in its circulation; but in healing by pus it is greatly retarded, or stagnant altogether.

Simple granulations are generally colourless; but those of three or four days' standing are moist, florid, and smooth; these form the connective tissue that supplies the part of the muscular tissue destroyed, mixed with a few fibres of elastic tissue. Again, granulations are sometimes arrested in their development; in these cases months may elapse without the cells developing. Again, in other cases the cells not only do not develop themselves, but degenerate, acquiring more the structure of pus cells; and it is in this condition they are found in the walls of sinuses, &c.; or they may lose all structure, and degenerate into a mass of molecular substances.

Fungus, or proud flesh, is granulations tinged with blood. These, again, may become inflamed, and purulent matter pervade the whole mass; all this retards the healing process. In wounds the pus serves as a cover; if it be thick and creamy, it should not be washed off; and when a wound heals, it has the power of contraction, at least the scab over it has. In granulation new blood-vessels form themselves; at first you will observe a bulging-out of the side of a neighbouring capillary, which prolongs itself to meet the same process of its neighbour, and as their blind ends meet they become absorbed: in this manner blood-vessels are supplied. Sometimes these bulgings burst and discharge their contents, consisting of red corpuscles; but these arrange themselves in one direction to meet the other dilatation on the opposite side, and at last are covered by a film which acts as a coat.

Secondary Adhesion.—This occurs whenever surfaces of wounds are well developed, but not covered by cuticle, and they are brought together.

In applying measures to produce this method of healing, certain circumstances are necessary, such as healthy granulations, &c. Healing under a scab is the most natural one, and requires no art whatever. It is termed cicatrix.

The scabs are formed from the fluid that exudes, therefore it has advantages over all others; but it is necessary to watch that no morbid exudation takes place under the scab; if so, you must remove it, but on no other account remove a scab. When a wound is nearly healed the scar contracts, and is bound firmly to the skin, but in old wounds the scar may be freely moved like the skin itself.

Fractures of Bone.

First, of the bones of the head. The jaw may be split owing to a fall, the split extending from the middle incisor to the neck of the bone, when the teeth will be loosened, with more or less bleeding. Should the skin be cut, it is termed compound fracture; if not cut, simple fracture. If the bone is shattered into many pieces, it is called comminuted; and should the soft structure be wounded as well, it is termed compound comminuted.

Treatment.—Remove the loose teeth, if any, and any pieces of bone that can be felt; and if the wound be too small to allow of this, enlarge it so that you can make a proper examination. The jaw must then be pressed together, and bandaged tightly, to prevent any friction; then give a dose of physic, which will nauseate the animal and prevent him from eating, as well as tend to keep down fever. The nourishment given afterwards must be composed of the best food, given in such a sloppy condition that the patient may drink or sip it, such as milk-bran, linseed gruels, oatmeal gruels, &c. With great care and attention there is nothing to prevent recovery.

In *Compound Fracture* you may perceive a dark fetid discharge from the wound; in a case of this kind you will require to inject a disinfectant, such as a solution of carbolic acid. If the edges of the bone are found to be carious, destroy this by injecting a solution of acid hydrochloric, one part to twenty of oil.

When the jaw is fractured, with displacement, you must get the parts into position; then stuff in tow bandages between the submaxillary spaces. Over this and surrounding the face a bandage must be applied, then a strap over this again to prevent movement. The mouth, of course, must be kept closed. Milk, however, can be given to support the patient.

For after-treatment apply soothing remedies, such as the solution of opium. Bathe frequently with warm water, and if fever sets in give aconite. Should there be occasion to extract the teeth, the hollows left are apt to become filled with food; so you must keep them clean by syringing with water after each meal. In old animals the healing process is very slow; it should therefore be considered whether or not the animal is worth the expense.

Treatment.—Cut down and remove the affected parts, if the bone be fractured; but if there be only thickening, and the skin not cut, apply some ung. hydrarg. beniod, to reduce the swelling.

You may also have fracture of the nasal bone. Sometimes this occurs high up, with depression, lessening the calibre of the nasal cavity, and causing the animal to roar when breathing. In a case of this kind you must raise the depression by means of a lever; or remove the offending bone, keeping the cavity clean, and watching for any inflammatory symptom.

Then, again, an animal may fall and fracture the orbital process of the frontal bone, causing total closure of the eyelids. There may or may not be a wound. If not, you must make one right over the arch. Then insert your lever, and endeavour to raise the parts; and as you do so, the eyelids will gradually open. If the bone is fractured into many pieces, clean and remove them, and then treat as a simple wound.

Fractures of the bones of the neck, back, pelvis, and limbs are as a rule attended with fatal consequences. In such cases there is generally little difficulty in arriving at a correct conclusion both as to the seat and cause of the inability of the animal to move; for the evidences presented soon leave little room for doubt, by showing that the animal has a broken back or a broken leg, as the case may be; therefore to enter into a description of these is scarcely necessary. All that is required is to be convinced that such is the case ere you order the animal to be slaughtered.

DISEASES OF THE EYE, Etc.

Gutta Serena.

In this disease the pupil becomes round, dilated, fixed, and insensible to light. In health, when the eye is exposed to a strong light it contracts, and in a weaker light it dilates; but in this complaint the eye is brighter than usual. It may attack one or both eyes, and may be partial or complete.

Causes.—Error in feeding; stomach-staggers; milk fever, &c. As a rule it is incurable; but if only arising from error in feeding, remove the cause and the effect will cease. Apply hot fomentations. Give a dose of physic and blister the cheek, &c., but if there is no change for the better after this treatment, you may abandon all hope.

Simple Ophthalmia

may be caused by a blow or common cold, or by any irritant that penetrates the organ of vision.

Symptoms.—Partial closing and swelling of the eyelids, with increased secretion of tears flowing down the cheeks, and corroding the skin with a kind of blue scum spreading over the whole extent of the eye.

Treatment.—Apply hot fomentations, and when

the swelling is very great, scarify the eyelids. Give also an aperient, applying likewise a weak solution of Goulard's Extract 1 ounce, tincture of opium 1 ounce, water 1 pint, and keep the animal in a dark place. There are many other diseases that the eye is liable to, into the respective symptoms and appearances of which it would perhaps be of little avail to enter; in such cases the help of a professional man is required in order to advise the best course to adopt. These diseases comprise cataracts, melanosis, fungus, hæmatodes, worms in the eye, tumours, &c., all of which require watchful care in their treatment, owing to the extreme delicacy of the organ affected.

Epizootic Aphthæ, or Foot-and-Mouth Disease.

When this disease first made its appearance in this country, it spread with alarming rapidity, and caused widespread consternation throughout the whole land; but now, owing to the well-directed vigilance of the Privy Council Veterinary Department, such devastation is scarcely possible. It affects all warm-blooded animals (but seldom attacks man or the horse), irrespective of class, colour, conformation, or age. It resembles to a certain extent small-pox, but differs in other particulars, for it will attack the same animal more than once. It may be defined as a febrile disease, sometimes involving the whole alimentary canal, the principal cause being contagion, while atmospheric influence has a great deal to do with it.

Symptoms.—The mouth is hot and tender, saliva dripping therefrom; partially chewed food is dropped, and the fetlocks are enlarged and painful. Vesicles appear along the mouth, which burst about twenty-four hours after their formation; and in milch-cows we have swelling of the udder and great tenderness, with vesicles. Few cases, however, when rightly managed, have much fever unless the udder is involved; in those cases where it is so, the secretion of milk is diminished, while the teats are so sore that they cannot be touched; if so, use the syphon. Again, it not unfrequently happens that the udder is left in a hard, indurated condition, and sometimes the teats slough off altogether.

Like other eruptive diseases, this one runs a prescribed course, which it generally accomplishes in fifteen days; anything that has a tendency to interrupt this course is injurious.

Treatment.—Allow soft sloppy food of an easily digestible nature, as the mouth, throat, and digestive organs are in an irritable condition. Opening medicine must be given if required, but great caution is to be exercised in its administration. The mouth should be washed out with a mild solution of alum. The feet, if hot and tender, should be bathed with tepid water, or placed in poultices; and if the vesicles have burst, apply cold water, with a mild astringent dressing; above all, cleanliness must be strictly enforced, or sloughing will set in. The udder, if hard, should be well fomented both before and after milking, and glycerine applied to the teats, while care should be taken not to allow the milk to accumulate. The disease as a rule only exhausts itself after invading the whole stock; therefore the healthy ought to be separated from the unhealthy animals, and disinfectants employed, the best being carbolic acid, as it possesses the power of destroying all organised life in putrefying solutions, while experiments have proved that virus loses its reproductive powers when exposed to its vapours, which can easily be accomplished. If you pour a little carbolic acid upon a red-hot coal or iron, it will penetrate everything within reach, and thus effectually destroy contagion.

Sanguineous Ascites, or Red-Water.

In Scotland this disease generally affects cows after calving, but in England and Ireland it occurs at any time, and at any age. When it affects cows after calving, the attack is often very acute, and reaches its climax in about three or four days. It is essentially a blood-disease, consisting in an alteration of its constituents; it is said that there is an abstraction of albumen and organic salts from the blood. The hæmatin or red colouring matter of the blood exudes through the coats, and becomes mixed with the urine.

The *Causes* which produce this state of matters are various. No doubt the vessels themselves are in a weakened or debilitated condition, but animals feeding on rank wet grass that is deficient in nutrient qualities may be predisposed to it. Some go so far as to say that frosted turnips will produce it. My own impression is that it is entirely due to poverty of the blood; for with poor blood we cannot expect a strong muscular system.

Symptoms are appetite and rumination suspended or irregular; also a gradual diminution of milk, which becomes thin, watery, and frothy. Urine at first of a pink colour, with increased quantity; diarrhœa, which gradually gives way to constipation; the urine becomes blacker and more blood-like; breathing greatly accelerated; the heart also is involved; ears and horns cold; animal gets weaker and weaker, and dies from sheer exhaustion.

Treatment.—In the first place, give one pound of Epsom salts; sulphur, quarter of a pound; croton oil, half a drachm, made up with treacle, one pound; follow this up with stimulants three or four times during the day, to which you can add ginger or gentian along with well-boiled gruel; allow the patient gentle exercise and as much good, pure, cold water as she can drink, with chlorate of potash, two ounces, dissolved in it.

Typhoid Fever in Calves.

This is comparatively a new disease, having only quite recently made its appearance. It was first observed near London, and attacks animals ranging from two to ten or twelve weeks old in a very abrupt and sudden manner. It is usually ushered in by diarrhœa. The patient becomes cold about the ears and extremities; the mouth hot; great prostration. In fact, the little sufferer cannot stand, the muscles of the body feeling soft and flabby; it lies with its head down; eyes dull and listless; sleeps a great deal; has no appetite and no thirst; the excretions become more and more affected. This state of matters gets gradually worse, and unless careful nursing is adopted, death will be the result in two days. Sometimes there is tympanitis and irritation of the bowels; at other times the lungs are affected, in which case there is frothing at the mouth, death soon occurring from suffocation.

Post-mortem Appearances. — Thin, dark, watery blood; moist, soft, and easily broken down, the body soon passes into a state of putrefaction. There are extravasation and patches of congestion on the fourth stomach and throughout the intestines; the liver and spleen are congested, while the lungs are engorged with dark-coloured blood. Lambs are also liable to this disease, and manifest the same symptoms as calves. Close, overcrowded places assist in its production, and in some instances the disease has been traced to the cow.

Treatment.—Although many calves perish, that is no reason why remedies should not be employed. Many people, however, are indifferent about the sufferings of a calf only a few weeks old, and care not how soon they are rid of the annoyance; therefore they will not be at the trouble to bestow a passing thought upon the patient, but allow it to linger on or die, as the case may be. Those, however, who are actuated by a humane desire to alleviate suffering, may proceed as follows with this disease:—As soon as you witness the first symptoms, give a small dose of castor-oil. If the patient is dull and listless, stimulants and tonics must be employed regularly and at short intervals, say every two hours. Administer two ounces of port-wine, with twenty or thirty drops of the liquor ammoniæ acetatis; or instead, one ounce of gin or whisky, with about eight ounces of newly drawn milk, every four hours. When the bowels are in a relaxed state, add about four ounces of lime-water.

Calves recover very slowly from this disease, and it is some time before they regain their usual appetite. When the milk appears to pass through undigested, well-boiled wheaten gruel may be given, sweetened with sugar or treacle. This remedy is of great service in white scour also.

An Eruptive Disease called Variola, or Smallpox.

This is a disease now of somewhat less interest than before the discovery of vaccination. It is of a very contagious nature, and is supposed to have been introduced into Europe from Asia. It is characterised by fever, with pustules appearing from the third to the fifth day, these suppurating from the eighth to the tenth. It possesses all the distinctive properties of the major exanthemata. It is capable of being produced by inoculation; and this inoculated smallpox communicates the disease as readily through the air as the natural smallpox, or that received without inoculation. Cowpox is, however, a very simple disease, and only affects the udder and teats. The bull also may become affected through inoculation. It is a malady that arises spontaneously in some cases, the causes being unknown. The symptoms are, first slight fever, with red blush on the udder and teats; this dies away, and is followed by patches of red, with a white spot in their centre. These continue two or three days, and then become hard and nodulated. The skin is now raised up in the form of vesicles, due to inflammation of the true skin; but this is soon relieved by effusion.

Treatment consists in keeping the animal comfortable, giving opening medicine, also applying fomentations to the udder and teats; in very severe cases poultice. The secretion of milk is not arrested; it may, however, be necessary to support the udder by a bandage. Give nitre in the water to drink, which will be all that is required.

Rinderpest, or Cattle Plague.

When this disease first made its appearance it spread rapidly over the country. It did not break out spontaneously, but was imported from abroad. The home of the disease seems to be the southern part of the Russian empire.

Some writers assert that it never arises spontaneously, but is an epizootic. This is an open question. It may be defined as an eruptive fever of a very contagious nature, due to some poison in the blood, the exact nature of which is not known. After the poison is introduced it remains latent for some time; this may vary from seven to eight days,—not less, however, than five, and never more than nine. During this period we have the poison gradually developing, when the symptoms begin to appear. First, there is a rise of the temperature of the body; this warmth soon gives way to coldness; in the course of two days we have an eruption taking place in the mouth and other parts, and on the fourth day the disease is fully developed. Appetite and rumination are entirely suspended; there is matter running from the eyes and nose; twitching of the muscles of the shoulder, accompanied by shivering and shaking of the head; the ears hang pendulous, feet drawn together, back arched, and altogether the animal has a very miserable and neglected appearance. As the malady advances the patient lies down and groans and coughs a good deal; in the latter stages diarrhœa sets in, which increases to dysentery, when death closes the scene. Sheep present much the same symptoms, when attacked, as cattle.

In almost all cases rinderpest is accompanied with liver-disease.

Treatment.—Everything has been tried for this disease, but with little success. Some practitioners recommend linseed-oil, turpentine, and opium—some one thing, and some another. It is always a very unwelcome visitor, and one that requires preventive measures to be strictly enforced, for in this course lies our security.

INDEX.

Abortion, 96.
Abscesses in the lungs, 70.
Aphtha, or thrush, 125.
Apoplexy, parturient, 100.
Arteries, diseases of the, 86.
Ascites, or dropsy, 47.
Atrophy of the heart, 85.
Biliary calculi, or gall-stones, 53.
Black leg, splenic apoplexy, black quarter, or quarter ill, 122.
Black quarter, quarter ill, black leg, or splenic apoplexy, 122.
Bladder, inflammation of the, or cystitis, 91.
Bladder, rupture of the, 94.
Bloody flux, or dysentery, 44.
Bloody urine, or hæmaturia, 91.
Bone, caries and necrosis of, 130.
Bone, diseases of the, 128.
Bone, fractures of, 157.
Bones, composition of the, 126.
Bowels, inflammation of the, or enteritis, 45.
Brain, water in the, or hydrocephalus, 118.
Bronchitis, or inflammation of the bronchial tubes, 62.
Burns and scalds, 151.
Caries and necrosis of bone, 130.
Catarrh, or common cold, 59.
Cattle-plague, or rinderpest, 168.
Choking, 14.
Chorea, or St. Vitus's Dance, 113.
Cold, common, or catarrh, 59.
Colic, 45.
Constipation, 42.
Cystitis, or inflammation of the bladder, 91.

Definition of disease, 9.
Degeneration, 54.
Description of diseases, 2.
Description of the intestines, 41.
Diabetes, 89.
Diarrhœa, 42.
Diarrhœa, white scour in calves, 43.
Digestion, diseases of the accessory organs of, 49.
Digestion, functional processes of, 4.
Dilatation of the heart, 84.
Diseases affecting the circulatory organs, 83.
Diseases after calving, 97.
Disease, definition of, 9.
Disease, description of, 2.
Diseases of the accessory organs of digestion, 49.
Diseases of the arteries, 86.
Diseases of the blood, 119.
Diseases of the bone, 128.
Diseases of the eye, 160.
Diseases of the generative organs, 92.
Diseases of the nervous system, 105.
Diseases of the organs of respiration, 56.
Diseases of the skin, 147.
Diseases of the urinary organs, 88.
Diseases of the veins, 87.
Dyspepsia in calves, 44.
Dropsy of the heart's bag, or hydrops pericarde, 84.
Dropsy, or ascites, 47.
Dropsy, ovarian, 93.
Dysentery, or bloody flux, 44.

INDEX.

Enchondroma, or tumour on the sternum or chest, 130.
Enteritis, or inflammation of the bowels, 45.
Epilepsy, or falling sickness, 115.
Epizootic aphthæ, or foot-and-mouth disease, 161.
Erysipelas, 120.
Eye, diseases of the, 160.
Falling sickness, or epilepsy, 115.
Fardel-bound, or impaction, 20.
Fatty degeneration of the heart, 86.
Fever, parturient, 97.
Foot-and-mouth disease, or epizootic aphthæ, 161.
Fractures of bone, 157.
Functional processes of digestion, 4.
Gall-stones, or biliary calculi, 53.
Gangrene, 11.
Giddiness, megrims, or vertigo, 114.
Glossanthrax, or carbuncle of the tongue, 124.
Glossitis, or inflammation of the tongue, 10.
Glossitis, the terminations of, 11.
Glossocele, or prolapsus linguæ, 13.
Grass staggers, 39.
Gutta serena, 160.
Hæmaturia, or bloody urine, 91.
Heart, atrophy of the, 85.
Heart, dilatation of the, 84.
Heart, fatty degeneration of the, 86.
Heart, hypertrophy of the, 85.
Heart, inflammation of the covering of the, or pericarditis, 83.
Heart, rupture of, 86.
Hepatitis, chronic, 51.
Hepatitis, or inflammation of the liver, 49.
Hoose in calves, 64.
Hydrocephalus, or water in the brain, 118.
Hydrops pericarde, or dropsy of the heart's bag, 84.
Hypertrophy of the heart, 85.

Hypertrophy, or chronic enlargement of the liver, 54.
Hysteria, 117.
Icterus, jaundice, or yellows, 52.
Impaction of the first stomach, 9.
Impaction, or fardel-bound, 20.
Inflammation, 23.
Inflammation, the terminations of, 32.
Intestines, description of the, 41.
Introduction, 1.
Jaundice, yellow, or icterus, 52.
Joints, open, 150.
Kidneys, inflammation of the, or nephritis, 90.
Larynx, inflammation of the, or laryngitis, 60.
Laryngitis, or inflammation of the larynx, 60.
Leucorrhœa, or the whites, 92.
Liver, chronic enlargement of the, or hypertrophy, 54.
Liver, inflammation of the, or hepatitis, 49.
Lock-jaw, or tetanus, 105.
Lungs, abscesses in the, 70.
Lungs, inflammation of the, or pneumonia, 67.
Lungs, structure of the, 66.
Mammitis, or inflammation of the udder, 103.
Megrims, vertigo, or giddiness, 114.
Mollities ossium, 129.
Necrosis, 131.
Nephritis, or inflammation of the kidneys, 90.
Ophthalmia, simple, 160.
Osteo-porosis, 129.
Osteo-sarcoma, or fleshy and bone tumour, 130.
Pancreas, the, 55.
Parturition, 94.
Pericarditis, or inflammation affecting the covering of the heart, 83.
Peritonitis, 47.
Pleuræ, inflammation of the, or pleurisy, 71.

INDEX.

Pleurisy, morbid changes of, 72.
Pleurisy, or inflammation of the pleuræ, 71.
Pleuro-pneumonia, 77.
Pneumonia, or inflammation of the lungs, 67.
Prolapsus ani and uteri, 48.
Prolapsus linguæ, or glossocele, 13.
Quarter ill, black leg, splenic apoplexy, or black quarter, 122.
Rachitis, 128.
Red-water, or sanguineous ascites, 163.
Respiration, diseases of the organs of, 56.
Rinderpest, or cattle plague, 168.
Ringworm, 148.
Rumination, 6.
Rupture of the heart, 86.
St. Vitus's dance, or chorea, 113.
Sanguineous ascites, or red-water, 162.
Scalds and burns, 151.
Skin, diseases of the, 147.
Smallpox, or variola, 167.
Spleen, the, 56.
Splenic apoplexy, black quarter, black ill, or black leg, 122.
Sternum or chest, tumour on the, or enchondroma, 130.
Stomach, distension of the first, tympanitis, or hoven, 17.
Stomach, impaction of the first, 9.
Stomach, the second, 20.
Structure of the lungs, 66.
Terminations of inflammation, the, 32.
Tetanus, or lock-jaw, 105.

Thrush, or aphthæ, 125.
Tissue, repair of, 152.
Tongue, carbuncle of the, or gloss-anthrax, 124.
Tongue, inflammation of the, or glossitis, 10.
Trachea, the, or windpipe, 61.
Tuberculosis, 81.
Tumour, fleshy and bone, or osteo-sarcoma, 130.
Tumours, 132.
Tumours, calcareous, 141.
Tumours, cartilaginous, or enchondromatis, 143.
Tumours, encysted, 142.
Tumours, fatty, 141.
Tumours, non-malignant, 137.
Tumours, melanotic, 143.
Tumours, scrofulous, 145.
Tympanitis, hoven, or distension of the first stomach, 17.
Typhoid fever in calves, 165.
Udder, inflammation of the, or mammitis, 103.
Urinary organs, diseases of the, 88.
Uterus or womb, inflammation of the, 93.
Uterus or womb, inversion of the, 93.
Variola, or smallpox, 167.
Veins, diseases of the, 87.
White scour in calves, diarrhœa, 43.
Whites, the, or leucorrhœa, 92.
Windpipe, the, or trachea, 61.
Wounds, 148.
Wounds, healing of, 153.

PRINTED BY BALLANTYNE, HANSON AND CO.
EDINBURGH AND LONDON.

www.ingramcontent.com/pod-product-compliance
Lightning Source LLC
Chambersburg PA
CBHW032153160426
43197CB00008B/896